Antimicrobial Chemotherapy

FIFTH EDITION

David Greenwood
Roger Finch
Peter Davey
Mark Wilcox

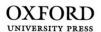

OXFORD
UNIVERSITY PRESS

OXFORD
UNIVERSITY PRESS

Great Clarendon Street, Oxford OX2 6DP

Oxford University Press is a department of the University of Oxford.
It furthers the University's objective of excellence in research, scholarship,
and education by publishing worldwide in

Oxford New York

Auckland Cape Town Dar es Salaam Hong Kong Karachi
Kuala Lumpur Madrid Melbourne Mexico City Nairobi
New Delhi Shanghai Taipei Toronto

With offices in

Argentina Austria Brazil Chile Czech Republic France Greece
Guatemala Hungary Italy Japan South Korea Poland Portugal
Singapore Switzerland Thailand Turkey Ukraine Vietnam

Oxford is a registered trade mark of Oxford University Press
in the UK and in certain other countries

Published in the United States
by Oxford University Press Inc., New York

© Oxford University Press, 2007

The moral rights of the author have been asserted

Database right Oxford University Press (maker)

First [edition] published by Ballière Tindall 1983
Second edition published 1989
Third edition published 1995
Fourth edition published 2000
Fifth edition published 2007
Reprinted 2008 (with correction)

A catalogue record for this title is available from the British Library

(Data available)

Library of Congress Cataloging in Publication Data

ISBN 978-0-19-857016-5

10 9 8 7 6 5 4 3 2

Typeset by Cepha Imaging Pvt Ltd., Bangalore, India.
Printed in Great Britain
on acid-free papèr by Ashford Colour Press Ltd, Gosport, Hampshire

Antimicrobial Chemotherapy

Preface

Almost everyone in the developed world will receive several courses of antibiotic during their lifetime. It is therefore not surprising that most clinicians and dentists will prescribe these drugs on a regular basis throughout their professional career. Indeed, several antibiotics figure among the most frequent of all prescribed drugs.

Antibiotics are not only life-saving with regard to severe infections, such as pneumonia, meningitis, and endocarditis, but are also responsible for controlling much of the morbidity associated with non-life-threatening infectious disease; illness is abbreviated, return to normal activities is hastened and there is often economic benefit to the individual, as well as society, by reducing the number of working days lost. In addition, infectious complications of many commonly conducted surgical procedures are now preventable by the use of peri-operative antibiotic prophylaxis. These benefits are well known to healthcare professionals and to the public who no longer fear infection in the way earlier generations did. The very success of antimicrobial chemotherapy has led to a perception that such agents are generally safe and that industry will continue to generate new agents to ensure the effective control of most infectious problems.

Antibiotics have largely been derived from natural sources, mainly from environmental bacteria and fungi. Their use in clinical medicine has been one of the major successes of the past century. The term 'antibiotic' was coined by Selman A Waksman, who recognized that these 'naturally derived substances were antagonistic to the growth of other micro-organisms in high dilution.' Over the years, other agents have been developed by chemical synthesis and more recently, as a result of genomic research. The term 'antimicrobial agents' captures all such compounds which in turn have been subdivided into antiviral, antibacterial, antifungal, antiparasitic (anthelminthic and antiprotozoal) agents according to the target pathogen. However, this purist approach is often ignored in practice and the term antibiotic is somewhat loosely applied to all these agents. The reader will find all such terms in use in this book.

Antibiotics are unique among therapeutic agents in that they target invading micro-organisms rather than any pathological process arising from host cells or tissues. Furthermore, unlike other classes of drug, micro-organisms have the inherent or acquired ability to evade or inactivate antimicrobial activity of these drugs. Such resistance presents a major threat to sustaining effective treatment of infectious disease.

Indeed, controlling antibiotic resistance is one of the greatest challenges facing healthcare professionals and the public and is likely to remain so. While new drugs, vaccines and better diagnostic methods are still a requirement, the fundamental issue is to ensure that existing agents are used effectively. This can only be achieved by ensuring that doctors, dentists, and, increasingly, other healthcare professionals who use these agents in the care of their patients, pursue good prescribing practice.

Good prescribing practice is the product of sound education, with particular emphasis on the acquisition of appropriate knowledge, skills, and professional behaviour. Good science informs good practice and since the knowledge base for prescribing practice is continuously expanding, the need for life-long learning is self-evident.

Patient safety remains paramount in medicine. Since antibiotics are often used in the management of mild to moderate community infections and the prophylaxis of infections this is of particular importance. The safety of antibiotics is monitored closely during drug development, at licensing and in clinical use. Since no drug is free from side effects, it is essential that the balance of risks and benefits of prescribing is appreciated and constantly considered by the prescribing practitioner. With more than 100 antimicrobial compounds currently available in the UK, this remains a particular challenge.

Setting forth the principles of rational antimicrobial chemotherapy is the whole purpose of this book. We sincerely hope that this 5th edition of *Antimicrobial Chemotherapy* will continue to furnish students and all healthcare professionals throughout the world with the necessary framework for understanding what antimicrobial agents will and will not do, and provide a firm basis for their informed use in the treatment and control of infection.

May 2006

D.G.
R.F.
P.D.
M.W.

Acknowledgements

The first edition of *Antimicrobial Chemotherapy* appeared in 1983, and was intended to bring to a wider audience elements of a very successful course (which still exists) taught at the University of Nottingham Medical School. The book was written by those who delivered the course and this tradition has continued through successive editions until the present one, when it was decided to invite expert colleagues from outside Nottingham, Peter Davey and Mark Wilcox, to join two of the original authors to consolidate and build on the growing success of the existing text.

The unique appeal of the book has always rested on its concern to introduce young doctors and other healthcare professionals to the principles that underpin the rational use of antibiotics in order to foster good habits of antimicrobial drug use. These principles are largely timeless, and, although the book had been extensively revised, some text written by other hands has inevitably been carried forward from edition to edition. We are therefore anxious to acknowledge these earlier contributions from our colleagues: Michael Emmerson, Patrick Greaves, William Irving (who also generously agreed to review chapters on antiviral agents for the present edition), Purvin Ispahani, Malcolm Lewis, the late Alastair Macrae, Francis O'Grady, Richard Slack, Kevin Towner, and Peter Wilkinson. Thanks are also due to Georgia Pinteau (and her predecessor, Helen Liepman), Clare Caruana and their colleagues at Oxford University Press for their unfailing courtesy, efficiency and patience during the gestation of the new edition.

Contents

Author biographies

David Greenwood DSc, PhD, FRCPath is Emeritus Professor of Antimicrobial Science at the University of Nottingham Medical School. Formerly at St Bartholomew's Hospital, London he has contributed over 200 books and articles on antimicrobial agents spanning 40 years, and in 1979 designed the very successful course on which this book was originally based.

Roger Finch FRCP, FRCP(Ed), FRCPath, FFPM is Professor of Infectious Diseases at the University of Nottingham Medical School. He has published over 300 books and articles, which include various aspects of antimicrobial chemotherapy. He is currently European Editor of *Current Opinion in Infectious Diseases* and formerly Editor-in-Chief of the *Journal of Antimicrobial Chemotherapy*. He is advisor to the UK Department of Health and European Centre for Disease Control.

Peter Davey MD, FRCP is Professor of Pharmacoeconomics at the University of Dundee and Honorary Consultant in Infectious Diseases, NHS Tayside. Formerly a Research Fellow at Tufts New England Medical Centre and the University of Birmingham he is currently President of the British Society for Antimicrobial Chemotherapy and has contributed over 200 books and articles on antimicrobial chemotherapy, pharmacoeconomics, and therapeutics.

Mark Wilcox, MRCPath, MD, is Professor of Medical Microbiology and Director of Infection Prevention and Control at the University of Leeds. He is a member of Council of the British Society for Antimicrobial Chemotherapy and an advisor to the UK Healthcare Commission, the Department of Health, and the Medicines and Healthcare Products Regulatory Agency. He has contributed over 200 books and articles on antimicrobial chemotherapy, medical microbiology and infection control.

Table 1 Some chemotherapeutic agents (and their indications) that predate the introduction of penicillin

Date	Agent	Disease/pathogen
Pre-1890	Extract of male fern	Tapeworm
	Santonin	Intestinal roundworm
	Oil of chenopodium	Intestinal roundworm
	Cinchona bark (quinine)	Malaria
	Ipecacuanha root (emetine)	Amoebic dysentery
	Mercury	Syphilis
	Chaulmoogra oil	Leprosy
Arsenicals and antimonials		
1905	Atoxyl	Trypanosomiasis
1909	Arsphenamine	Syphilis
1912	Neoarsphenamine	Syphilis
1912	Tartar emetic	Leishmaniasis
1917	Tartar emetic	Schistosomiasis
1919	Tryparsamide	Trypanosomiasis
Dyes and dye derivatives		
1891	Methylene blue	Malaria
1904	Trypan red	Trypanosomiasis
1906	Trypan blue	Trypanosomiasis
1916	Suramin	Trypanosomiasis[a]
1926	Plasmochin	Malaria
1932	Mepacrine	Malaria (etc.)
1932	Prontosil red	Bacteria
1934	Chloroquine[b]	Malaria
Other substances		
1895	Hexamine	Bacteria (urine)
1899	Pyocyanase	Bacteria (topical)
1925	Tetrachloroethylene	Hookworm
1939	Tyrothricin	Bacteria (topical)

[a]Later (1940s) also used in onchocerciasis.

[b]Chloroquine was first synthesized in 1934 in Germany, but developed in the USA in 1945.

the concept of antibiosis and its therapeutic potential was not new. In fact, moulds had been used empirically in folk remedies for infected wounds for centuries and the observation that organisms, including fungi, sometimes produced substances capable of preventing the growth of others was as old as bacteriology itself. One antibiotic substance, pyocyanase, produced by the bacterium *Pseudomonas aeruginosa*, had actually been used therapeutically by instillation into wounds, at the turn of the twentieth century.

Thus, when Alexander Fleming interrupted a holiday to visit his laboratory in St Mary's Hospital in early September 1928 to make his famous observation on a contaminated culture plate of staphylococci, he was merely one in a long line of workers who had noticed similar phenomena. However, it was Fleming's observation that sparked off the events that led to the development of penicillin as the first antibiotic in the strict sense of the term.

The actual circumstances of Fleming's discovery have become interwoven with myth and legend. Attempts to reproduce the phenomenon have led to the conclusion that the lysis of staphylococci in the area surrounding a contaminant *Penicillium* colony on Fleming's original plate could have arisen only by an extraordinary concatenation of accidental events, including the vagaries of temperature of an English summer.

Early attempts to exploit penicillin foundered, partly through a failure to purify and concentrate the substance. Fleming made some attempts to use crude filtrates in superficial infections and there is documentary evidence that Cecil George Paine, a former student of Fleming's, successfully treated gonococcal ophthalmia with filtrates of *Penicillium* cultures in Sheffield as early as 1930. However, it was left to Ernst Chain, a German refugee who had been recommended to Florey as a biochemist, to obtain a stable extract of penicillin. Chain had been set the task of investigating naturally occurring antibacterial substances (including lysozyme, another of Fleming's discoveries) as a biochemical exercise. It was with his crude extracts that the first experiments were performed in mice and men. Since these extracts contained less than 1% pure penicillin, it is fortunate that problems of serious toxicity were not encountered.

Further development of penicillin was beyond the means of wartime Britain, and Florey visited the USA in 1941 with his assistant, Norman Heatley, to enlist the support of the American authorities and drug firms. Once Florey had convinced them of the potential of penicillin, progress was rapid and by the end of the Second World War bulk production of penicillin was in progress and the drug was beginning to become readily available.

Cephalosporins

The discovery of the cephalosporins (which are structurally related to the penicillins) is equally extraordinary. Between 1945 and 1948, Giuseppe Brotzu, former Rector of the University of Cagliari, Sardinia, investigated the microbial flora of a sewage outflow in the hope of discovering naturally occurring antibiotic substances. One of the organisms recovered from the sewage was a *Cephalosporium* mould that displayed striking inhibitory activity against several bacterial species—including *Salmonella typhi*, the cause of typhoid and now considered as a serotype of *S. enterica*—that were beyond the reach of penicillin at that time. Brotzu carried out some preliminary bacteriological and clinical studies, and published some encouraging results in a local house journal. However, he lacked the facilities to develop the compound further, and nothing more might have been heard of the work if he had not sent a reprint of his paper to a British acquaintance, Dr Blyth Brooke, who drew it to the attention of the Medical Research Council in London. They advised contacting Howard Florey, and Brotzu sent the mould to the Sir William Dunn School in 1948.

The first thing to be discovered by the Oxford scientists was that the mould produced two antibiotics, which they called cephalosporin P and cephalosporin N, because the former inhibited Gram-positive organisms (e.g. staphylococci and streptococci), whereas the latter was active against Gram-negative organisms (e.g. *Escherichia coli* and *S. typhi)*. Neither of these substances is a cephalosporin in the sense that the term is used today: cephalosporin P proved to be an antibiotic with a steroid-like structure, and cephalosporin N turned out to be a penicillin (adicillin). The forerunner of the cephalosporins now in use, cephalosporin C, was detected later as a minor component on fractionation of cephalosporin N. Such a substance could easily have been dismissed, but it was pursued because it exhibited some attractive properties, notably stability to the enzymes produced by some strains of staphylococci that were by then threatening the effectiveness of penicillin.

Antibiotics from soil

The development of penicillin, cephalosporin C, and, subsequently, their numerous derivatives represents only one branch of the antibiotic story. The other main route came through an investigation into antimicrobial substances produced by micro-organisms in soil. The chief moving spirit was Selman A. Waksman, an emigré from the Russian Ukraine, who had taken up the study of soil microbiology in the USA as a young man. In 1940, Waksman initiated a systematic search for non-toxic antibiotics produced by soil micro-organisms, notably actinomycetes, a group that includes the *Streptomyces* species that were to yield many therapeutically useful compounds. Waksman was probably influenced in his decision to undertake this study by the first reports of penicillin and by the discovery by an ex-pupil, René Dubos, of the antibiotic complex tyrothricin in culture filtrates of *Bacillus brevis*.

Waksman's first discoveries were, like Dubos's tyrothricin, too toxic for systemic use, although they included actinomycin, a compound later used in cancer chemotherapy. The real breakthrough came in 1943 with the discovery by Waksman's research student, Albert Schatz, of streptomycin, the first aminoglycoside antibiotic, which was found to have a spectrum of activity that neatly complemented penicillin by inhibiting many Gram-negative bacilli and—very importantly at that time—*Mycobacterium tuberculosis*. It remained the staple treatment for tuberculosis (together with some synthetic compounds; see below) until the antibiotic rifampicin—named after the 1955 French gangster film *Rififi*—was introduced in 1968.

The success of streptomycin stimulated the pharmaceutical houses to join the chase in the years following the end of the Second World War. Soil samples by the hundred thousand from all over the world were screened for antibiotic-producing micro-organisms. Thousands of antibiotic substances were discovered and rediscovered and, although most failed preliminary toxicity tests, by the mid-1950s representatives of most of the major families of antibiotics including aminoglycosides, chloramphenicol, tetracyclines, and macrolides, had been found.

Since 1960 few truly novel antibiotics have been discovered, although a surprising number of naturally occurring molecular variations on the penicillin structure have emerged. A more fruitful approach, especially with penicillins and cephalosporins, has been to modify existing agents chemically in order to derive semisynthetic compounds with improved properties.

Non-antibiotic antibacterial compounds

Alongside developments in naturally occurring antibiotics, chemists and microbiologists have also been successful in seeking synthetic chemicals with antibacterial activity. Most have emerged through an indefinable mixture of biochemical know-how and luck rather than the rational targeting of vulnerable processes within the microbial cell.

The first important advance came with the discovery of *para*-aminosalicylic acid and isoniazid as effective antituberculosis drugs in the early 1950s, ushering in the era of reliable triple therapy (with streptomycin) for tuberculosis. Among the rest, the nitrofurans have a long history stretching back to before the Second World War, but attracted little attention until the development of nitrofurantoin in the early 1950s. The diaminopyrimidine, trimethoprim, was first synthesized in America by George Hitchings and his colleagues in 1956.

Commercially the most successful synthetic antibacterial agents have been the quinolones. The original compound, nalidixic acid, discovered in the 1960s as a by-product of the synthesis of the antimalarial agent chloroquine, was of minor importance, but after an unpromising start quinolones began to assume a more significant role in the 1980s when derivatives such as norfloxacin and ciprofloxacin emerged that exhibited much better activity against a broader spectrum of bacteria.

Antifungal, antiparasitic, and antiviral agents

The revolution in therapy brought about by the numerous antibacterial 'wonder drugs' was not mirrored in infections caused by other microbes, but considerable progress in the treatment of non-bacterial infection was nevertheless made in the second half of the twentieth century.

Treatment of fungal infections was the first to benefit. In 1949 at the height of the search for naturally occurring antibacterial compounds, Elizabeth Hazen and Rachel Brown discovered an antibiotic with surprisingly good antifungal activity. They named it nystatin after the New York State Department of Health in whose laboratories they worked. The related polyene, amphotericin B, was developed by scientists at Squibb in the 1950s. Another antifungal antibiotic, griseofulvin, had been described as early as 1939, but not used in human medicine until 1958, following the work by James Gentles in Glasgow on dermatophyte infections in experimental animals. A major step forward occurred in the 1970s with the discovery in Germany and Belgium of the unexpectedly broad-spectrum antifungal activity of certain nitroimidazole derivatives such as clotrimazole and ketoconazole (which offered the added advantage that it could be given orally) leading to the later development of the triazoles, fluconazole and itraconazole.

Among antiprotozoal agents, most progress was made among antimalarial agents, starting with the development in America after the Second World War of a pre-war German discovery, chloroquine, and culminating in the successful testing of artemisinin, the active ingredient of an ancient Chinese herbal remedy qinghaosu in the late 1970s. Many other protozoal diseases fared less well, but patients suffering from amoebic dysentery, giardiasis, and trichomonal vaginitis (and those with infections caused by anaerobic bacteria) benefited from the development in France around 1960 of metronidazole, a synthetic compound based on the structure of a naturally-occurring antibiotic, azomycin.

Even helminthic disease treatment was to profit from the intense research activity, albeit through investigations into drugs for worm infections of farm animals. Remarkably, by the early 1980s, three anthelminthic compounds—praziquantel, albendazole, and ivermectin—were available, which between them offered safe and effective treatment for a diverse range of human worm infections.

For many years, antimicrobial agents played a very minor part in the treatment of viral infections, although prevention of a number of viral diseases through the use of vaccines was outstandingly effective. The first real breakthrough came with the nucleoside analogue aciclovir as an offshoot of anticancer research in the mid-1970s. Even this drug, the first antiviral agent to display selective toxicity, was restricted to the treatment of herpesvirus infections. Antiviral chemotherapy was not to come of age for another decade, when the emerging AIDS pandemic stimulated the pharmaceutical industry into a flurry of activity that has produced an array of drugs offering palliative if not curative therapy.

The discovery of the first 'miracle drugs' was sanguinely declared by some to herald the virtual conquest of infection. More than 60 years of use have prompted a more sober assessment of the limitations of antimicrobial therapy. Microbes have shown amazing versatility in avoiding, withstanding, or repelling the antibiotic onslaught, while parallel medical advances have provided a large and increasing group of vulnerable patients for them to attack. Antimicrobial agents are essential tools of modern medicine, but the battle against infection is far from won. The challenge now is to preserve the remarkable achievements of the twentieth century by learning to use these powerful drugs more judiciously.

Part 1

General properties of antimicrobial agents

Chapter 1

Inhibitors of bacterial cell wall synthesis

The essence of antimicrobial chemotherapy is selective toxicity—to kill or inhibit the microbe without harming the patient. So far as bacteria are concerned, a prime target for such an attack is the cell wall, since practically all bacteria (with the exception of mycoplasmas) have a cell wall, whereas mammalian cells lack this feature. Several groups of antibiotics, notably β-lactam agents (penicillins, cephalosporins, and their relatives) and glycopeptides (vancomycin and teicoplanin) take advantage of this difference. A few less important antibiotics also act at this level and some compounds used in the treatment of tuberculosis and leprosy act on the specialized mycobacterial cell wall (p. 66).

In general bacterial cell walls conform to two basic patterns, which can be distinguished by that most familiar of all microbiological techniques, the Gram stain. Gram-positive (staphylococci, streptococci, etc.) and Gram-negative (escherichia, pseudomonas, klebsiella, etc.) bacteria respond differently to cell wall active agents and it is helpful to understand the basis for this difference.

Cell wall construction

In both Gram-positive and Gram-negative bacteria the cell wall is formed from a cross-linked chain of alternating units of N-acetylglucosamine and N-acetylmuramic acid, known as peptidoglycan or mucopeptide. The process of synthesis is illustrated in outline in Fig. 1.1. N-acetylmuramic acid is manufactured from N-acetylglucosamine by the addition of lactic acid derived from phosphoenolpyruvate. Three amino acids are then added to form a muramic acid tripeptide. Meanwhile, two D-alanine residues, produced from L-alanine by an enzyme called alanine racemase, are joined together by another enzyme, D-alanine synthetase. The linked unit, D-ala-D-ala, is added to the tripeptide and the muramic acid pentapeptide thus formed is joined to an N-acetylglucosamine molecule and passed to a lipid carrier in the cell membrane. The whole building block is transported

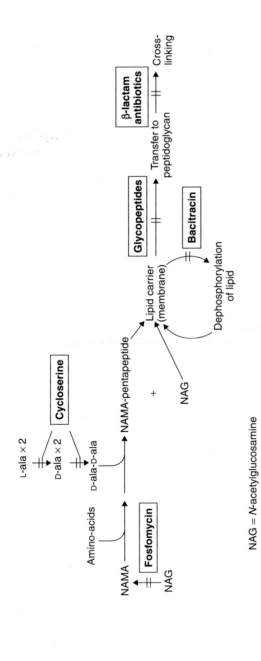

Fig. 1.1 Simplified scheme of bacterial cell wall synthesis showing site of action of cell wall-active antibiotics. (Reproduced from *Medical Microbiology*, 16th Edition by David Greenwood (2003), with permission from Elsevier.

across the cell membrane and added to the end of the existing cell wall. Finally, adjacent units are cross-linked to give the wall its strength.

In Gram-positive organisms the cell wall structure is thick (about 30 nm), tightly cross-linked, and interspersed with polysugarphosphates (teichoic acids), some of which have a lipophilic tail buried in the cell membrane (lipoteichoic acids). Gram-negative bacteria, in contrast, have a relatively thin (2–3 nm), loosely cross-linked peptidoglycan layer and no teichoic acid.

External to the Gram-negative peptidoglycan is a membrane-like structure, composed chiefly of lipopolysaccharide and lipoprotein, which prevents large molecules such as glycopeptides from entering the cell. Small hydrophilic molecules enter Gram-negative bacilli through aqueous channels—called porins—within the outer membrane. Differential activity among some groups of antibiotics, notably the penicillins and cephalosporins, is influenced by their ability to negotiate these porin channels and this, in turn, reflects the size and ionic charge of substituents carried by the individual agents.

β-Lactam antibiotics

Penicillins, cephalosporins, and certain other antibiotics belong to a family of compounds, collectively known as β-lactam antibiotics, which share the structural feature of a β-lactam ring. In the penicillins the β-lactam ring is fused to a five-membered thiazolidine ring, whereas the cephalosporins display a fused β-lactam/dihydrothiazine ring structure (Fig. 1.2). The β-lactam ring is the Achilles' heel of this group of antibiotics because many bacteria possess enzymes (β-lactamases; see p. 130) that are capable of breaking open the ring and rendering the molecule antibacterially inactive.

Penicillins

The original preparations of penicillin were found on analysis to be mixtures of four closely related compounds that were called penicillin F, G, K, and X. Benzylpenicillin (penicillin G), often simply called 'penicillin', was chosen for further development because it exhibited the most attractive properties and because a manufacturing process was developed in which *Penicillium chrysogenum* was persuaded to produce benzylpenicillin almost exclusively.

Early attempts to modify this structure relied on presenting the *Penicillium* mould used to produce penicillin with different side-chain precursors during the manufacturing process. Later a method was discovered of removing the side-chain of benzylpenicillin to liberate the penicillin nucleus, 6-amino-penicillanic acid (6-APA). Various chemical groupings could then be added to

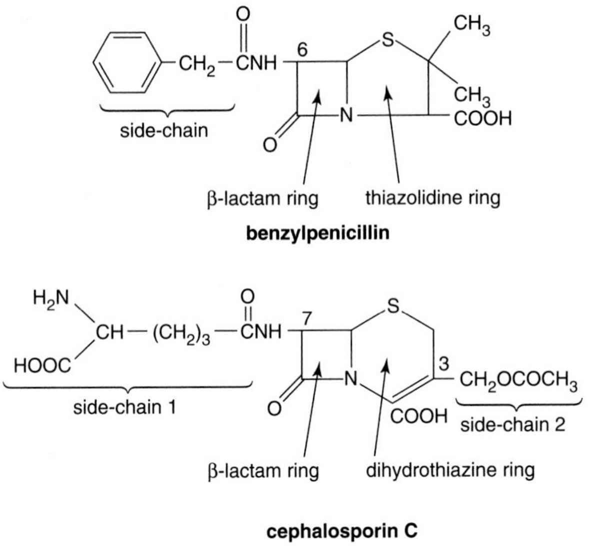

Fig. 1.2 Structures of benzylpenicillin and cephalosporin C, forerunners of the penicillin and cephalosporin groups, respectively. The fused-ring systems and the side-chains, which offer the possibility of modifications introduced in semi-synthetic derivatives, are indicated.

6-APA according to the ingenuity of the chemist; a large number of compounds, collectively called semisynthetic penicillins, have been prepared in this way.

Benzylpenicillin revolutionized the treatment of many potentially lethal bacterial infections, such as scarlet fever, puerperal sepsis, bacterial endocarditis, pneumococcal pneumonia, staphylococcal sepsis, meningococcal meningitis, gonorrhoea, syphilis (and other spirochaetal diseases), anthrax, and many anaerobic infections. The overwhelming importance of benzylpenicillin as a major breakthrough in therapy may be gauged from the fact that it remains today the treatment of choice for all these diseases.

However, resistance has eroded the value of benzylpenicillin. Nearly all staphylococci and many strains of gonococci are now resistant. Moreover, pneumococci exhibiting reduced susceptibility to benzylpenicillin are increasingly prevalent. Such strains are of two types: those for which the minimum inhibitory concentration (MIC) of benzylpenicillin is increased from the usual value of about 0.02 mg/l to 0.1–1 mg/l, and those for which the MIC exceeds 1 mg/l. The former are sufficiently sensitive to enable the antibiotic to be successfully used in high dosage, except in pneumococcal meningitis.

Cephalosporins

Cephalosporins generally exhibit a somewhat broader spectrum than penicillins, though, idiosyncratically, they lack activity against enterococci. They are mostly stable to staphylococcal β-lactamase and lack cross-allergenicity with penicillins (see p. 221).

The original cephalosporin, cephalosporin C, was never marketed, but has given rise to a large family of compounds that continues to expand. The extra carbon atom in the fused ring (Fig. 1.2), offers the possibility of modifications at the carbon designated C-3 (right-hand side of the molecule in Fig. 1.2). Consequently, there are many more cephalosporins than penicillins (Table 1.2). Alterations at either end of the molecule may profoundly affect antibacterial activity but, as a generalization, substituents at the C-3 position have more influence on pharmacokinetic properties. Certain cephalosporins such as cefalotin (no longer widely available) and cefotaxime have an acetoxymethyl side chain at C-3 which is slowly altered by liver enzymes. The altered cephalosporin is usually less active than the parent antibiotic and may display altered pharmacokinetic behaviour, but there is little evidence that the clinical effectiveness is impaired. Several cephalosporins, including cefamandole, cefotetan, cefmenoxime, cefopera-zone, and the oxa-cephem latamoxef possess a complex side-chain at the C-3 position that has been implicated in haematological side effects in some patients (see p. 228).

The earliest cephalosporins, cefalotin and cefaloridine, are not absorbed when given orally. Moreover, it soon became clear that the Gram-negative organisms within their spectrum were capable of elaborating a wide variety of enzymes that exhibited potent cephalosporinase activity (see pp. 130–134). As with penicillins, developments within the cephalosporin family were aimed at devising compounds with more attractive properties: oral absorption or other improved pharmacological properties; stability to inactivating enzymes; better intrinsic activity; or a combination of these features.

Cephalosporins are commonly described as first, second, third, or even fourth generation compounds. These loose terms, which are best avoided, refer to:

- early compounds such as cefalotin and cefalexin that were available before about 1975 (first generation);
- β-lactamase stable compounds such as cefuroxime and cefoxitin (second generation);
- compounds such as cefotaxime that combine β-lactamase stability with improved intrinsic activity (third generation);

Table 1.2 Categorization of cephalosporins in clinical use

Parenteral compounds			Oral compounds		
Cefalotin	Cefacetrile	Ceforanide	Cefalexin[a]	Cefaloglycin	Cefroxadine
Cefaloridine	Cefapirin	Cefonicid	Cefradine[a]	Cefadroxil[a]	Cefatrizine
Cefazolin	Cefazedone	Ceftezole	Cefaclor[a]	Cefprozil[a]	Loracarbef[b]
Cefamandole					

Compounds with improved β-lactamase stability			Compounds with improved β-lactamase stability		
			Non-esterified	*Esterified*	
Cefuroxime[a]	Cefmetazole	Cefotiam	Cefixime[a]	Cefuroxime axetil[a]	
Cefoxitin	Cefotetan	Cefminox	Ceftibuten	Cefpodoxime proxetil[a]	
			Cefdinir	Cefetamet pivoxil	
				Cefteram pivoxil	

Compounds with improved intrinsic activity and β-lactamase stability					
Cefotaxime[a]	Cefmenoxime	Latamoxef[c]		Cefotiam hexetil	
Ceftriaxone[a]	Ceftizoxime	Flomoxef[c]		Cefditoren pivoxil	
Cefodizime	Cefuzonam			Cefcapene pivoxil	

Compounds distinguished by activity against *Pseudomonas aeruginosa*

Broad spectrum	Medium spectrum	Narrow spectrum
Ceftazidime[a]	Cefoperazone	Cefsulodin
Cefpirome[a]	Cefpimizole	
Cefepime	Cefpiramide	

[a]Compound available in the UK (2006).

[b]Strictly a carbacephem.

[c]Strictly oxa-cephems.

◆ a group of newer compounds that the manufacturers would like to persuade us have special properties (fourth generation).

In fact, the cephalosporins display such diverse properties that they defy any rigid categorization, but it is helpful to distinguish between those (the majority) that have to be administered parenterally and those that can be given orally. Among injectable compounds, it is useful to consider separately those with improved β-lactamase stability and those notable for their antipseudomonal activity (Table 1.2).

Parenteral compounds susceptible to enterobacterial β-lactamases

Cephalosporins in this group are of limited clinical value and have been largely superseded by other derivatives; all have been abandoned in the UK. Cefazolin has the unusual property of being excreted in fairly high concentration in bile; cefamandole exhibits a modestly expanded spectrum. Others, including cefapirin, ceforanide, and cefonicid, offer no discernible advantage over earlier congeners such as cefalotin.

Parenteral compounds with improved β-lactamase stability

An important advance was achieved with the development of cephalosporins that exhibit almost complete stability to the common β-lactamases of enterobacteria such as *Esch. coli* and *Klebsiella aerogenes*. The first of these were cefuroxime and cefoxitin, the latter being one of a group of cephalosporins, collectively called cephamycins, which have a β-lactam ring modified by the addition of a stabilizing methoxy substituent. Other cephamycins available in some countries include cefotetan, cefmetazole, and cefminox. The cephamycins are unusual in displaying useful activity against anaerobes of the *Bacteroides fragilis* group.

These compounds have been overshadowed by the appearance of cephalosporins that combine almost complete stability to most β-lactamases with much improved intrinsic activity. Cefotaxime was the forerunner of this group of compounds, but several others are available: ceftizoxime and cefmenoxime are similar to cefotaxime; ceftriaxone displays a sufficiently long plasma half-life to warrant once-daily administration; cefodizime is said to possess immunomodulating properties.

Latamoxef (moxalactam), which is strictly an oxa-cephem (see below), also displays activity analogous to that of cefotaxime and its relatives, but differs in possessing useful activity against *B. fragilis* and related anaerobes. However, latamoxef has lost favour owing to toxicity problems and it is no longer widely available.

Compounds distinguished by antipseudomonal activity

Ps. aeruginosa is not susceptible to most cephalosporins and, as with penicillins, considerable efforts have been made to find derivatives that include this important opportunist pathogen in their spectrum. Ceftazidime, cefpirome, and cefepime add activity against *Ps. aeruginosa* to broad-spectrum activity comparable with that of cefotaxime and its congeners. These compounds have established a useful role in the management of *Ps. aeruginosa* infections in seriously ill patients. However, the antistaphylococcal activity is suspect and cefpirome may have some advantage in this respect. Cefepime retains activity against some opportunist Gram-negative bacilli that develop resistance to cefotaxime and its relatives.

Among other antipseudomonal cephalosporins, cefoperazone, cefpimizole, and cefpiramide are not distinguished by any unusual activity against other organisms and cefsulodin is extraordinary in being virtually inactive against bacteria other than *Ps. aeruginosa*.

Oral cephalosporins

Early development of the cephalosporins yielded cefalexin, a compound of modest activity, particularly in terms of its bactericidal action against Gram-negative bacilli, but which is virtually completely absorbed when given orally. Many other oral derivatives are structurally minor variations on the cefalexin theme. Such compounds include cefradine (the properties of which are indistinguishable from those of cefalexin), cefaclor (which is more active against the important respiratory pathogen *H. influenzae*), cefadroxil (which exhibits a modestly extended plasma half-life) and cefprozil (which exhibits improved intrinsic activity). Loracarbef is a carbacephem (carbon replacing sulphur in the fused-ring structure), but is otherwise structurally identical to cefaclor. Not surprisingly, its properties closely resemble those of cefaclor.

Cefixime and ceftibuten are structurally unrelated to cefalexin. They display much improved activity against most Gram-negative bacilli, but at the expense of antistaphylococcal (and, in the case of ceftibuten, antipneumococcal) activity, which is very poor. Another compound of this type, cefdinir, appears to lack these defects.

The principle of esterification to produce pro-drugs with improved oral absorption has also been applied to cephalosporins. Two such compounds, cefuroxime axetil and cefpodoxime proxetil, are available in the UK; cefteram pivoxil, cefetamet pivoxil, cefotiam hexetil, cefditoren pivoxil, and cefcapene pivoxil are marketed elsewhere. These esters are fairly well absorbed by the oral route and deliver the parent drug into the bloodstream. Cefpodoxime, cefteram, and cefetamet are more active than the others against most organisms within the spectrum, although cefetamet has poor activity against staphylococci.

A summary of the antimicrobial spectrum of the most important cephalosporins is presented in Table 1.3.

Cephalosporins: prescriber's survival kit

- *Cefuroxime*: good broad-spectrum work-horse (cefuroxime axetil for oral use)
- *Cefotaxime/ceftriaxone*: more active than cefuroxime; save for serious infections
- *Ceftazidime*: serious pseudomonas infections only; injectable
- *Cefalexin/cefradine/cefaclor*: oral absorption their chief virtue

Other β-lactam agents

In addition to penicillins and cephalosporins, various other compounds display a β-lactam ring in their structure (Fig. 1.3). The cephamycins, the oxa-cephems latamoxef and flomoxef, and the carbacephem loracarbef—all of which share the general properties of cephalosporins—are examples of such structural variants. Fundamentally different are clavulanic acid, a naturally occurring substance obtained from *Streptomyces clavuligerus*, and two penicillanic acid sulphones, sulbactam and tazobactam. These compounds have little useful antibacterial activity, but act as β-lactamase inhibitors. They are used in combination with β-lactamase-labile agents with a view to restoring their activity. Partner compounds reflect the manufacturer's interests: clavulanic acid is combined with amoxicillin (co-amoxiclav) or ticarcillin; sulbactam with ampicillin; and tazobactam with piperacillin.

Structurally novel compounds that exhibit antibacterial activity in their own right include the carbapenems (imipenem, meropenem, panipenem, and ertapenem) and aztreonam, one of a group of compounds, collectively known as monobactams, which have a β-lactam ring but no associated fused-ring system.

The carbapenems are stable to most bacterial β-lactamases, and exhibit the broadest spectrum of all β-lactam antibiotics, with high activity against nearly all Gram-positive and Gram-negative bacteria other than intracellular bacteria such as chlamydiae. Imipenem is readily hydrolysed by a dehydropeptidase located in the mammalian kidney and is administered

Table 1.3 Summary of the spectrum of antibacterial activity of cephalosporins available in the UK (2006)

Cephalosporin	Staphylococci	Streptococci[a]	Neisseria spp.	Haemophilus influenzae	Enterobacteria	Pseudomonas aeruginosa	Bacteroides spp.
Cefuroxime	Good	Very good	Good	Good	Good	–	–
Cefotaxime Ceftriaxone	Good	Very good	Very good	Very good	Very good	Poor	Poor
Ceftazidime	Fair	Good	Very good	Very good	Very good	Good	Poor
Cefpirome	Good	Very good	Very good	Very good	Very good	Good	–
Cefalexin Cefradine Cefadroxil	Good	Good	Poor	Poor	Variable	–	–
Cefaclor	Good	Good	Fair	Good	Variable	–	–
Cefixime	Poor	Very good	Good	Good	Very good	–	–
Cefprozil	Good	Good	Very good	Very good	Very good	–	–
Cefpodoxime	Good	Very good	Very good	Good	Very good	–	–

–, no useful activity. [a]Enterococci are resistant to all cephalosporins.

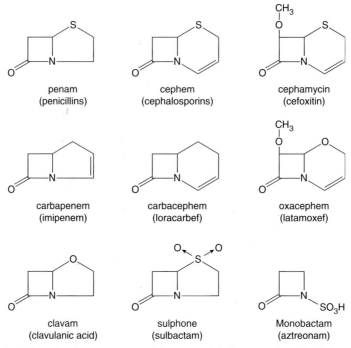

Fig. 1.3 Basic molecular structures of β-lactam antibiotics currently available (examples in parentheses).

together with a dehydropeptidase inhibitor, cilastatin. Aztreonam is also β-lactamase stable, but, in contrast to carbapenems, the activity is restricted to aerobic Gram-negative bacteria.

Factors affecting β-lactam agents

Penicillins and other β-lactam antibiotics are categorized as bactericidal agents, but this is true only when bacteria are actively dividing. Moreover, the way bacteria respond to β-lactam antibiotics is affected by subtle differences in the mode of action. Several other features of the response that may sometimes have therapeutic implications have also been discovered.

Mode of action of β-lactam agents

All β-lactam antibiotics interfere with the final cross-linking reaction that gives the cell wall its strength (Fig. 1.1). However, several forms of the enzyme that performs this reaction are needed to maintain the complex molecular architecture of the cell and these are differentially inhibited by various β-lactam agents. These target enzymes belong to a group of proteins to which penicillin and other β-lactam antibiotics bind (penicillin-binding proteins; PBPs). *Esch. coli*, the best-studied species, has seven of these proteins, numbered la, lb, 2, 3, 4, 5, and 6 in order of decreasing molecular weight. PBPs 4–6 are thought to be unconnected with the antibacterial effect of β-lactam agents, since mutants lacking these proteins do not seem to be disabled in any way. Binding to the remainder has been correlated with the various morphological effects of β-lactam antibiotics on Gram-negative bacilli. Thus, cefalexin and its close congeners, as well as aztreonam, bind almost exclusively to PBP 3 and inhibit the division process, causing the bacteria to grow as long filaments. The amidinopenicillin, mecillinam, binds preferentially to PBP 2 and causes a generalized effect on the cell wall so that the bacteria gradually assume a spherical shape. Most other β-lactam antibiotics bind to PBPs 1–3 and, in sufficient concentration, induce the formation of osmotically fragile, wall-deficient forms (called spheroplasts), which typically emerge at the cell wall growth site as the cell starts to divide. The morphological events are illustrated in Fig. 1.4. An important consequence of differences in binding is that compounds such as cefalexin, aztreonam, and mecillinam, which bind only to PBP 3 or PBP 2, are much more slowly bactericidal to Gram-negative bacilli that those that bind PBPs 1, 2, and 3.

In Gram-negative bacilli, rupture of spheroplasts can be quantitatively prevented by raising the osmolality of the growth medium, so cell death appears to be an osmotic phenomenon. The lethal event in Gram-positive organisms, which have much thicker cell walls, appears to be autolysis triggered by the release of lipoteichoic acid following exposure to β-lactam antibiotics.

Optimal dosage effect

A further complication in Gram-positive organisms is that increasing the concentration of β-lactam antibiotics often results in a reduced bactericidal effect. The mechanism of this effect (known as the Eagle phenomenon after its discoverer) is obscure, but may be related to the multiple sites of penicillin action and the fact that cell death occurs only during active growth: saturating a relatively insusceptible penicillin-binding protein may rapidly halt growth and thereby prevent the lethal events that normally follow inhibition of another PBP by lower drug levels.

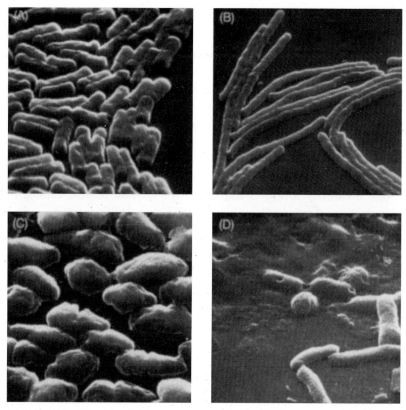

Fig. 1.4 Morphological effects of penicillins and cephalosporins on Gram-negative bacilli (scanning electron micrographs): (A) Normal *Esch. coli* cells; (B) *Esch. coli* exposed to cefalexin, 32 mg/l, for 1 h; (C) *Esch. coli* exposed to mecillinam, 10 mg/l, for 2 h; (D) *Esch. coli* exposed to ampicillin, 64 mg/l, for 1 h, showing lysed debris, central wall lesions, and a spheroplast; higher concentrations of most β-lactam antibiotics cause this effect. (A–C from Greenwood D, O'Grady F, *Journal of Infectious Diseases*, 1973; **128**: 791–4; D from Greenwood D, O'Grady F, *Journal of Medical Microbiology*, 1969; **2**: 435–41.)

Persisters and penicillin tolerance

In both Gram-positive and Gram-negative bacteria, a proportion of the population, called persisters, survive exposure to concentrations of β-lactam antibiotics lethal to the rest of the culture. They remain dormant so long as the antibiotic is present and resume growth when it is removed. In addition, some strains of staphylococci and streptococci display 'tolerance' to β-lactam antibiotics in that they succumb much more slowly than usual to the lethal action of β-lactam agents. The therapeutic significance, if any, of persisters is unknown, but penicillin tolerance has been implicated in therapeutic failures in bacterial endocarditis where bactericidal activity is crucial to the success of treatment (p. 318).

Postantibiotic effect

Much has also been made of laboratory observations that the antimicrobial activity of β-lactam agents may persist for an hour or more after the drug is removed. This effect is not confined to β-lactam agents and is more consistently demonstrated with Gram-positive than with Gram-negative organisms. Theoretically, knowledge of postantibiotic effects might influence the design of dosage regimens, but in practice they are too erratic to be used in this way, even if the laboratory observations could be convincingly shown to have clinical relevance, which is presently not the case.

Glycopeptides   For staphs and streps; use mainly for MRSA

The glycopeptides vancomycin and teicoplanin are complex heterocyclic molecules consisting of a multi-peptide backbone to which are attached various substituted sugars. These compounds bind to acyl-D-alanyl-D-alanine in peptidoglycan, thereby preventing the addition of new building blocks to the growing cell wall (Fig. 1.1). Glycopeptides are too bulky to penetrate the external membrane of Gram-negative bacteria, so the spectrum of activity is virtually restricted to Gram-positive organisms. Acquired resistance used to be uncommon, but resistant strains of enterococci are now widely prevalent and staphylococci exhibiting reduced susceptibility are causing concern. Avoparcin, a glycopeptide formerly used in animal husbandry (now banned in the European Union), has been implicated in generating resistance in enterococci, but human use of glycopeptides is equally important. Some Gram-positive genera, including *Lactobacillus* spp., *Pediococcus* spp., and *Leuconostoc* spp. are inherently resistant to glycopeptides, but these organisms are seldom implicated in disease.

Vancomycin

This antibiotic is widely used for the treatment of infections caused by staphylococci that are resistant to methicillin and other β-lactam antibiotics, and for serious infections with Gram-positive organisms in patients who are allergic to penicillin. It is poorly absorbed when given by mouth and must be given by injection. Oral administration is indicated in the treatment of antibiotic-associated diarrhoea caused by toxigenic strains of *Clostridium difficile* (p. 302–3), but such use is discouraged because of the fear of undermining the value of this compound by promoting the emergence of resistance in Gram-positive cocci.

Early preparations of vancomycin contained impurities that gave the drug a reputation for toxicity. The purified formulations now available are much safer, but renal and ototoxicity still occur, particularly with high dosage. The drug is given by slow intravenous infusion to avoid 'red man syndrome' (p. 220).

Teicoplanin

This is a naturally occurring mixture of several closely related compounds with a spectrum of activity similar to that of vancomycin, although some coagulase-negative staphylococci (*Staphylococcus epidermidis* etc.) are less susceptible to teicoplanin. Some strains of enterococci that are resistant to vancomycin (those with the VanB phenotype; p. 138–140) retain susceptibility to teicoplanin. Unlike vancomycin, teicoplanin can be administered by intramuscular injection; it also has a much longer plasma half-life than vancomycin and a reduced propensity to cause adverse reactions.

Other cell wall active agents

Bacitracin Topical use only

Bacitracin is a cyclic peptide antibiotic, made up of about 10 amino acids joined in a ring. It was first obtained from a strain of *Bacillus subtilis* grown from the infected wound of a 7-year-old girl, Margaret Tracy, in whose honour the antibiotic was named.

The spectrum of activity of bacitracin and related cyclic peptides such as gramicidin and tyrocidine is restricted to Gram-positive organisms. They are too toxic for systemic use but are found in topical preparations. Bacitracin also finds a place in microbiology laboratories in the presumptive identification of *Streptococcus pyogenes*, which is exquisitely susceptible to its action. Bacitracin acts by preventing regeneration of the lipid carrier in the cell membrane, which is left in an unusable phosphorylated form after transporting cell wall subunits (Fig. 1.1).

Cycloserine Tuberculosis only

Cycloserine has broad-spectrum, but rather feeble antibacterial activity. It is now used only against multiresistant *Mycobacterium tuberculosis* (p. 349). The drug bears a structural resemblance to the D-isomer of alanine and inhibits alanine racemase. It also blocks the synthetase enzyme that links two D-ala molecules together before they are inserted into the cell wall (Fig. 1.1). Antituberculosis agents that act on special features of the mycobacterial cell wall are discussed in Chapter 3.

Fosfomycin   **Uncomplicated cystitis only**

Fosfomycin (Fig. 1.5) is a naturally occurring antibiotic originally obtained from a species of *Streptomyces* isolated in Spain. It is formulated as the sodium salt for parenteral use, but this is unsuitable for oral administration. It is well tolerated, and the ready emergence of bacterial resistance that is observed in vitro does not appear to have been a major problem in treatment. The trometamol (tromethamine) salt, which is highly soluble, well absorbed, and excreted in high concentration in urine, is preferable to the calcium salt for oral therapy. Although fosfomycin is used for assorted purposes in some countries, it is not sufficiently reliable for serious infections. It is best reserved for uncomplicated cystitis, for which the trometamol salt is well suited.

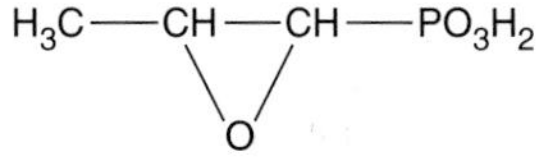

$$H_3C\text{---}CH\text{---}CH\text{---}PO_3H_2$$
$$\diagdown O \diagup$$

Fig. 1.5 Structure of fosfomycin.

Fosfomycin inhibits the pyruvyl transferase enzyme that brings about the condensation of phosphoenolpyruvate and *N*-acetylglucosamine in the formation of *N*-acetylmuramic acid (Fig. 1.1). Gram-positive cocci are less susceptible than Gram-negative rods. The precise level of activity is a matter of dispute, since the in-vitro activity can be manipulated by altering the test medium. Glucose-6-phosphate potentiates the activity against many Gram-negative bacilli by inducing the active transport of fosfomycin into the bacterial cell.

Chapter 2

Inhibitors of bacterial protein synthesis

The remarkable process by which proteins are manufactured on the ribosomal conveyor belt according to a blueprint provided by the cell nucleus is so fundamentally important and intrinsically fascinating that no one who has studied any aspect of modern biology can fail to have encountered it. Although the general mechanism is thought to be universal, the process as it occurs in bacterial cells is sufficiently different from mammalian protein synthesis to offer scope for the selective toxicity required of therapeutically useful antimicrobial agents. The chief difference involves the actual structure of the ribosomal workshop in both protein and RNA components.

In order to understand how the various inhibitors of protein synthesis work it is helpful to be aware of the main features of the process. The first step is the formation of an initiation complex, consisting of messenger RNA (mRNA), transcribed from the appropriate area of a DNA strand; the two ribosomal subunits; and methionyl transfer RNA (tRNA) (*N*-formylated in bacteria) which occupies the 'peptidyl donor' site (P site) on the larger ribosomal subunit. Aminoacyl tRNA appropriate to the next codon to be read slots into place in the aminoacyl 'acceptor' site (A site), and an enzyme called peptidyl transferase attaches the methionine to the new amino acid with the formation of a peptide bond. The mRNA and the ribosome now move with respect to one another so that the dipeptide is translocated from the A to the P site and the next codon of the mRNA is aligned with the A site in readiness for the next aminoacyl tRNA. The process continues to build up amino acids in the nascent peptide chain according to the order dictated by mRNA until a 'nonsense' codon is encountered, which signals chain termination.

The selective activity of therapeutically useful inhibitors of protein synthesis is far from absolute. Some, such as tetracyclines and clindamycin, have sufficient activity against eukaryotic ribosomes to be of value against certain protozoa. Moreover, the mitochondria of mammalian and other eukaryotic cells (which may have been derived from endosymbiotic bacteria during the course of evolution) carry out protein synthesis that is susceptible to some antibiotics used in therapy. The selectivity of these antibiotics is, therefore, a product not only of structural differences in the ribosomal targets, but also of access to, and affinity for, those targets.

Inhibitors of bacterial protein synthesis with sufficient selectivity to be useful in human therapy include aminoglycosides, chloramphenicol, tetracyclines, fusidic acid, macrolides, lincosamides, streptogramins, oxazolidinones, and mupirocin.

Aminoglycosides

Classification

The first aminoglycoside, streptomycin, discovered in 1943 (see Historical introduction), was later found to be just one of a large family of related antibiotics produced by various species of *Streptomyces* and *Micromonospora*. Aminoglycosides derived from the latter genus, such as gentamicin, are distinguished in their spelling by an 'i' rather than a 'y' in the 'mycin' suffix.

Structurally, most aminoglycosides consist of a linked ring system composed of aminosugars and an aminosubstituted cyclic polyalcohol (aminocyclitol). One antibiotic usually included with the group, spectinomycin, contains no aminoglycoside substituent and is properly regarded as a pure aminocyclitol.

The aminocyclitol moiety of most aminoglycosides consists of one of two derivatives of streptamine: streptidine (present in streptomycin and its relatives) or deoxystreptamine (present in most other therapeutically useful aminoglycosides) (Fig. 2.1). Deoxystreptamine-containing aminoglycosides can, in their turn, be subdivided into two major groups: the neomycin group and the kanamycin group. The aminoglycosides most commonly used in medicine, including gentamicin and tobramycin, belong to the kanamycin group. The designation 'kanamycin', 'gentamicin', or 'neomycin' indicates a family of closely related compounds and commercial preparations usually contain a mixture of these. For example, gentamicin, as used therapeutically, is a mixture of several structural variants of the gentamicin C complex (Fig. 2.2).

General properties

The aminoglycosides are potent, broad-spectrum bactericidal agents that are very poorly absorbed when given orally and are therefore administered by injection. The spectrum includes most Gram-negative bacilli and staphylococci. They lack useful activity against streptococci and anaerobes, but the activity against streptococci can often be improved by using them in

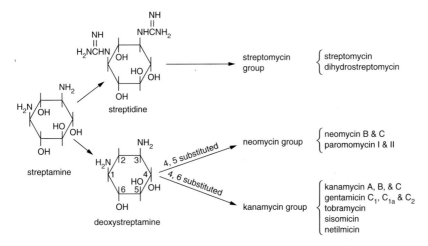

Fig. 2.1 Grouping of therapeutically useful aminoglycosides according to characteristics of the aminocyclitol ring. In most aminoglycosides the aminocyclitol moiety is either streptidine or deoxystreptamine, both derivatives of streptamine. The deoxystreptamine group can be subdivided into those in which sugar substituents are linked at the 4- and 5-hydroxyls, and those substituted at the 4- and 6-hydroxyl positions.

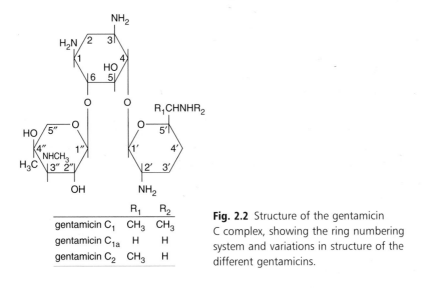

	R₁	R₂
gentamicin C_1	CH_3	CH_3
gentamicin C_{1a}	H	H
gentamicin C_2	CH_3	H

Fig. 2.2 Structure of the gentamicin C complex, showing the ring numbering system and variations in structure of the different gentamicins.

conjunction with penicillins, with which they interact synergically. Aminoglycosides penetrate poorly into mammalian cells and are of limited value in infections caused by intracellular bacteria. Some members of the group display important activity against *Mycobacterium tuberculosis* or

Pseudomonas aeruginosa. All of them display considerable toxicity affecting both the ear and the kidney (Table 2.1).

Aminoglycoside assay

Because of their toxicity use of aminoglycosides requires careful laboratory monitoring to make sure that plasma concentrations are adequate, but not so high that toxic levels are reached. Assays should be performed if treatment is for longer than 48 h, particularly if there is any renal impairment, and always in older patients. Indeed it might be considered negligent if a patient developed side effects attributable to aminoglycoside therapy and the drug concentration had not been monitored.

The therapeutic range of concentrations of aminoglycosides such as gentamicin in plasma was originally thought to be 2–10 mg/l, but it is far from certain that single high peak concentrations correlate simply with adverse effects. Indeed, it is now common to use once-daily aminoglycoside therapy, which requires doses that achieve relatively high peak concentrations. Such regimens have been shown to be as safe as conventional multidose therapy and what may be more important is the 'area under the curve', i.e. the total concentration of drug related to time. Thus, relatively minor increases in pre-dose 'trough' levels, such as occur with minimal renal impairment, may be of greater relevance than high peaks.

Mode of action

Streptomycin binds to a particular ribosomal protein and a single amino acid change in this protein results in streptomycin resistance. Aminoglycosides of the kanamycin and neomycin groups bind at a different site and are generally unaffected. Several effects of the binding of streptomycin and other aminoglycosides have been noted, including a tendency to cause misreading of certain codons of mRNA resulting in the production of defective proteins, some of which may affect membrane integrity. Other evidence suggests that the primary site of action lies in the formation of non-functioning initiation complexes, or inhibition of the translocation step in polypeptide synthesis. None of these hypotheses fully explains the potent bactericidal activity of aminoglycosides compared with other inhibitors of protein synthesis. Definitive solutions to these and other paradoxical aspects of aminoglycoside action are still the subject of dispute.

Aminoglycosides enter bacteria by an active transport process involving respiratory quinones. These are absent in streptococci and anaerobes which are consequently resistant.

Table 2.1 Summary of the antibacterial spectrum and toxicity of some aminoglycosides

Aminoglycoside	Activity against:					Relative degrees of:	
	Staphylococci	Streptococci	Enterobacteria	*Pseudomonas aeruginosa*	*Mycobacterium tuberculosis*	Ototoxicity	Nephrotoxicity
Streptomycin	Good	Poor	Good	Poor	Good	+++	+
Kanamycin	Good	Poor	Good	Poor	Good	++	++
Gentamicin	Good	Fair	Good	Good	Poor	++	++
Tobramycin	Good	Poor	Good	Good	Poor	++	++
Netilmicin	Good	Poor	Good	Good	Poor	+	+
Amikacin	Good	Poor	Good	Good	Good	++	+
Neomycin	Good	Poor	Good	Poor	Fair	+++	+++

Streptomycin   `Mainly tuberculosis`

The use of streptomycin has declined with the appearance of other aminoglycosides, although it is still a component of several antituberculosis regimens recommended by the World Health Organization (see Chapter 25). It is also used in the treatment of some rarer conditions, including plague, brucellosis, bartonellosis, and tularaemia, possibly for want of adequate evidence that more modern agents might be effective.

Neomycin group

Neomycin is the most ototoxic of the aminoglycosides and it is now little used, except in topical preparations; even this use is discouraged because of the risk of promoting the emergence of aminoglycoside resistance. It has also been given orally together with other agents to sterilize the gut before abdominal surgery, but the inactivity of aminoglycosides against anaerobes ensures that most of the gut flora escapes, and the procedure is not without risk of systemic toxicity. Framycetin, a common component of topical preparations, is identical to neomycin B.

One aminoglycoside of the neomycin group, paromomycin, is unusual in exhibiting activity against the protozoa causing amoebic dysentery and leishmaniasis as well as some tapeworms. However, other drugs are preferred in the treatment of these parasitic diseases (see Chapter 5).

Kanamycin group

Important members of this large group include kanamycin itself, gentamicin, tobramycin, netilmicin, and a semisynthetic derivative of kanamycin A, amikacin.

In its naturally occurring form kanamycin is a mixture of three closely related compounds, kanamycin A, B, and C. Pharmaceutical preparations consist almost exclusively of kanamycin A, although kanamycin B (bekanamycin) is available in some countries. The spectrum of activity is similar to that of streptomycin (and includes *M. tuberculosis*), but it retains activity against streptomycin-resistant strains and is less likely to cause vestibular damage.

Kanamycin has largely been superseded by gentamicin and tobramycin (deoxykanamycin B), which are more active against many enterobacteria and, more importantly, include *Ps. aeruginosa* in their spectrum. This has been a major factor in the popularity of these agents for the 'blind' therapy of serious infection before the results of laboratory tests are known. The relative merits of gentamicin and tobramycin have been the subject of much debate.

Ps. aeruginosa (Table 2.2). Resistance is common among staphylococci, but less so in streptococci. However, resistant *Streptococcus pyogenes* strains are increasing in prevalence.

Macrolides have many attractive properties as well-tolerated oral compounds that display good tissue penetration. Their spectrum of activity makes them particularly suitable for the treatment of respiratory and soft-tissue disease and for infections caused by susceptible intracellular bacteria. They are also used in campylobacter enteritis if the severity of infection warrants antimicrobial treatment, and in *Legionella pneumophila* pneumonia.

Erythromycin

Erythromycin, the oldest and most widely used macrolide antibiotic, was discovered at a time when resistance of staphylococci to penicillin was first becoming a serious problem. In the fear that its usefulness might be similarly compromised, it was at first used as a reserve antistaphylococcal agent or for streptococcal infections in patients allergic to penicillin.

Erythromycin base is broken down in the acid conditions of the stomach and it is administered in the form of enteric-coated tablets that protect the antibiotic until it reaches the absorption site in the duodenum. Alternatively, the stearate salt or esterified pro-drug forms are used for oral administration. Two ester formulations are in general use: the ethylsuccinate and the estolate. Erythromycin lactobionate and erythromycin gluceptate are available for intravenous use. The estolate is generally regarded as the most toxic formulation because of its propensity to cause reversible cholestatic jaundice. However, this uncommon complication can arise with any of the preparations. Erythromycin is liable to cause nausea and abdominal cramps and this has diminished its popularity.

Erythromycin derivatives

Efforts to modify the properties of erythromycin have been more successful in generating compounds with improved pharmacological features rather than enhanced antibacterial activity. Much interest has centred on altering the molecule in such a way that the reactive groups responsible for the acid lability are modified. Such changes increase the bioavailability and often extend the plasma half-life. Any improvement in antibacterial activity is generally modest, but enhanced tissue penetration may render these compounds more effective. Acid-stable derivatives of erythromycin also appear to be less prone to cause gastrointestinal upset. Macrolides of this type include azithromycin, clarithromycin, dirithromycin, and roxithromycin.

Azithromycin

In this semisynthetic macrolide, a nitrogen atom has been inserted into the lactone ring of erythromycin to produce a 15-membered ring structure that is described as an azalide. Azithromycin has a considerably improved bioavailability and a much extended plasma half-life compared with erythromycin. The antibacterial spectrum is similar to that of erythromycin, although it is somewhat more active against some important respiratory pathogens such as *H. influenzae* and *L. pneumophila;* there is also some improvement in activity against enteric Gram-negative bacilli, but this is unlikely to be of therapeutic benefit.

The most important property of azithromycin is the long terminal half-life, which enables it to be administered once a day. A single dose is effective in chlamydial and gonococcal infections of the genital tract.

Clarithromycin

This derivative of erythromycin is altered in the body to yield a metabolite that retains antibacterial activity, but has altered pharmacokinetic properties. The activities of clarithromycin and its metabolite are similar to that of erythromycin, although concentrations required to inhibit legionellae and chlamydiae are generally lower.

There have been claims of much enhanced penetration into pulmonary sites, beneficial interactions between the parent compound and the metabolite, and other minor advantages. It is doubtful whether these translate into significantly improved therapeutic efficacy, but clarithromycin is better absorbed and less prone to cause abdominal discomfort than earlier macrolides. It has been successfully used in combination regimens for the treatment of infections with *Helicobacter pylori* and some mycobacteria, notably those of the *M. avium* group.

Dirithromycin

Dirithromycin is slightly less active than erythromycin against most organisms within the spectrum, but it has a much extended plasma half-life and has been successfully used for once-daily treatment of respiratory tract, skin, and soft tissue infections.

Roxithromycin

Roxithromycin is another erythromycin derivative and, not surprisingly, exhibits activity very similar to the older drug. It differs, however, in having an extended plasma half-life, a feature that may be related to extensive binding to plasma proteins.

Ketolides

A new class of erythromycin derivatives, the ketolides, has been obtained by introducing a keto function into the macrolactone ring of erythromycin after removal of one of the sugars. These compounds share the Gram-positive spectrum of the earlier macrolides, but retain activity against macrolide-resistant strains.

The only compound of this type presently available is telithromycin. A similar compound, cethromycin, is under development at the time of writing.

Other macrolides

Other macrolides that have been used in various parts of the world include oleandomycin (or its better absorbed derivative triacetyloleandomycin) and a series of compounds with a 16-membered ring, including spiramycin, josamycin, midecamycin, kitasamycin, and rokitamycin. None of them seems to offer much therapeutic advantage over erythromycin. Spiramycin is sometimes used as an alternative to pyrimethamine in infections caused by the protozoan parasite, *Toxoplasma gondii*.

Lincosamides   Staphylococcal and anaerobic infection

The original lincosamide, lincomycin, a naturally occurring product of *Streptomyces lincolnensis*, has been superseded by clindamycin (7-chloro-7-deoxylincomycin; Fig. 2.7), which exhibits improved antibacterial activity.

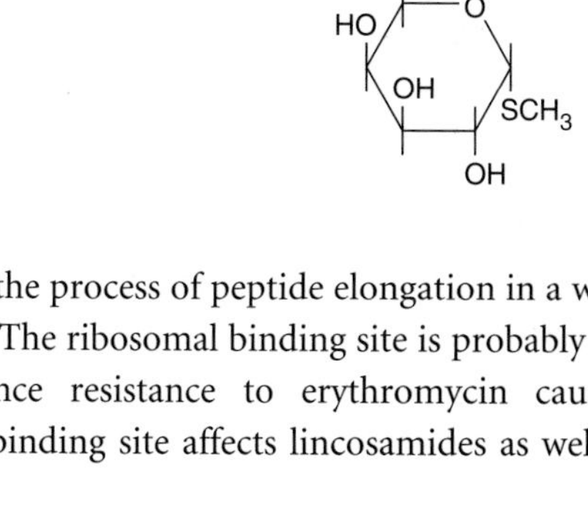

Fig. 2.7 Structure of clindamycin.

Lincosamides interfere with the process of peptide elongation in a way that has not been precisely defined. The ribosomal binding site is probably similar to that of erythromycin, since resistance to erythromycin caused by methylation of the ribosomal binding site affects lincosamides as well.

Lincomycin and clindamycin possess good antistaphylococcal and antistreptococcal activity and have also proved therapeutically useful in the treatment of infections due to *Bacteroides fragilis* and some other anaerobes. Enterobacteria and *Ps. aeruginosa* lie outside the spectrum of activity (Table 2.2). Clindamycin exhibits some activity against parasitic protozoa and has been used in toxoplasmosis, malaria, and babesiosis.

Clindamycin hydrochloride, like chloramphenicol, is extremely bitter. For oral administration the drug is formulated in capsules or as the biologically inactive palmitate, which liberates the parent compound in vivo. Clindamycin phosphate, the soluble form used for intravenous administration, is similarly inactive in the test-tube, but is hydrolysed to the active drug in the body.

Patients treated with clindamycin (or lincomycin) commonly experience diarrhoea caused by a clostridial toxin, which occasionally develops into a potentially fatal pseudomembranous colitis (see p. 224). Other antibiotics, notably ampicillin and broad-spectrum cephalosporins, may also cause this side effect, but the incidence of toxin-associated colitis appears to be somewhat higher following clindamycin therapy.

Streptogramins

Each member of the streptogramin family is not one antibiotic, but two: they are produced as synergic mixtures by various species of *Streptomyces*. One of these compounds, virginiamycin, has been extensively used as a growth promoter in animal husbandry. Another streptogramin, pristinamycin, is sometimes used as an antistaphylococcal agent in Continental Europe, but plasma concentrations after oral administration do not greatly exceed inhibitory levels and solubility problems have militated against parenteral use. A formulation consisting of the water-soluble derivatives, quinupristin and dalfopristin, is, however, suitable for infusion and is now preferred for human therapy.

The two components of streptogramin antibiotics are structurally different. Alone they exhibit feeble bacteristatic activity, but in combination the effect is bactericidal. Component A is a polyunsaturated peptolide that causes distortion of the aminoacyl-tRNA binding site, hindering further growth of the peptide chain. The action of component B, a hexadepsipeptide, is less well understood, but it is proposed that it binds to an adjacent site and that the combined effect is to constrict the channel through which the nascent peptide is extruded from the ribosome. Protein synthesis is completely blocked and the consequences are lethal to the bacterial cell.

The activity of streptogramins is virtually restricted to Gram-positive organisms. Their major claim to attention is that they retain activity against multiresistant staphylococci and some enterococci, notably *Enterococcus faecium*. Unfortunately, *E. faecalis*, which is more commonly encountered, is often resistant.

Mupirocin Topical use only

Mupirocin (formerly known as pseudomonic acid) is a component of the antibiotic complex produced by the bacterium *Ps. fluorescens*. The novel structure consists of monic acid with a short fatty acid side-chain (Fig. 2.8). The terminal portion of the molecule distal to the fatty acid resembles isoleucine, and mupirocin inhibits protein synthesis by blocking incorporation of the amino acid into polypeptides. The analogous process in mammalian cells is unaffected.

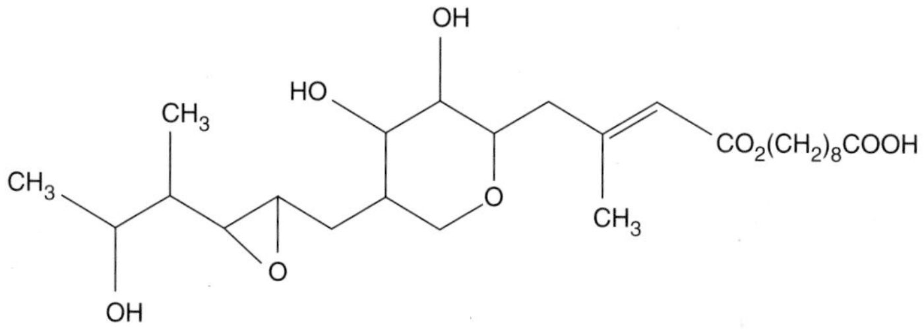

Fig. 2.8 Structure of mupirocin.

The spectrum of activity embraces staphylococci and streptococci, but excludes most enteric Gram-negative bacilli (Table 2.2). Hopes that mupirocin might be useful in systemic therapy were thwarted by the realization that the compound is inactivated in the body. Consequently, its use is restricted to topical preparations. Mupirocin has proved particularly useful in the eradication of staphylococci from nasal carriage sites.

Oxazolidinones For multiresistant staphylococci and streptococci

Several oxazolidinones have attracted attention over the years owing to their activity against Gram-positive organisms, including staphylococci, pneumococci, and enterococci. They are well absorbed by the oral route and exhibit bacteristatic activity. They act at an early stage in protein synthesis by blocking the formation of the 70 S initiation complex. A principal attraction of these compounds is that they do not show cross-resistance to other classes of drugs.

The most widely investigated member of the family, linezolid, has been available for several years. Early indications are that it is safe and effective and it appears to be a useful reserve agent in patients infected with multiresistant strains of staphylococci or other Gram-positive cocci. The drug is active against *M. tuberculosis* and there is some evidence that it might be useful in infections with drug-resistant strains. The chief limitation of linezolid is an effect on bone marrow cells that largely limits the length of treatment to 2 weeks.

Inhibitors of protein synthesis: prescriber's survival kit

- *Gentamicin*: good all purpose aminoglycoside for serious infections (remember streptococci, anaerobes, and intracellular organisms are not covered; monitor plasma levels)
- *Amikacin*: reserve for organisms resistant to gentamicin
- *Doxycycline*: good standby for infections where tetracyclines appropriate
- *Erythromycin*: useful oral antistaphylcoccal/antistreptococcal agent
- *Azithromycin*: effectiveness in a single dose makes it attractive for chlamydial infections to ensure compliance

Chapter 3

Synthetic antibacterial agents and miscellaneous antibiotics

Various targets other than the cell wall and ribosome are open to attack by chemotherapeutic agents. This chapter describes the properties of inhibitors of bacterial nucleic acid synthesis, compounds that act on the bacterial cell membrane, and agents used solely for the treatment of mycobacterial disease. Many of these compounds are synthetic chemicals rather than antibiotics in the strict sense.

Inhibitors of nucleic acid synthesis

Given the universality of nucleic acid as the basis of life, it is surprising that so many antimicrobial agents have been discovered that selectively interfere with the functions of DNA and RNA. Some, like the sulphonamides and diaminopyrimidines, achieve their effect indirectly by interrupting metabolic pathways that lead to the manufacture of nucleic acids; others, of which the quinolones and nitroimidazoles are prime examples, exert a more direct action.

Sulphonamides Mostly obsolete

The discovery of Prontosil in the 1930s was a major breakthrough in the chemotherapy of bacterial infections (see Historical introduction). Activity of the dye is due to the liberation in the body of sulphanilamide, an analogue of *para*-aminobenzoic acid (Fig. 3.1), which is essential for bacterial folate synthesis. Most bacteria synthesize folic acid and cannot take it up preformed from the environment. Mammalian cells, in contrast, use preformed folate and cannot make their own. Sulphonamides block an early stage in folate synthesis leading to various effects, including a failure to synthesize purine nucleotides and thymidine. Chemical modification of the sulphanilamide molecule has resulted in the production of hundreds of different sulphonamides, which differ chiefly in their pharmacological properties.

Sulphonamides have a broad antibacterial spectrum, though the activity against enterococci, *Pseudomonas aeruginosa*, and anaerobes is poor. They are predominantly bacteriostatic, and relatively slow to act: several generations of

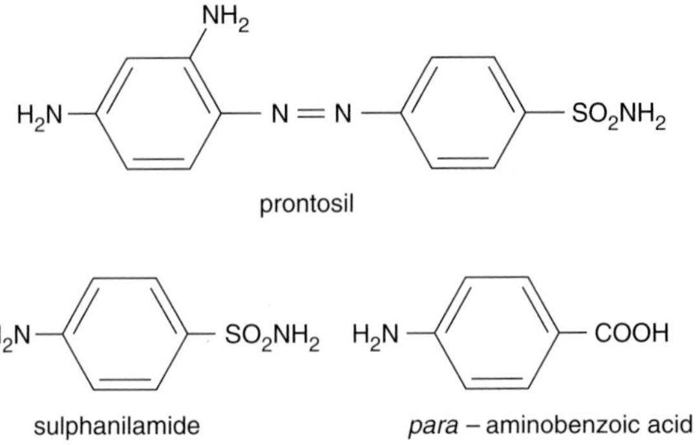

Fig. 3.1 Structures of prontosil, sulphanilimide, and p-aminobenzoic acid.

bacterial growth are needed to deplete the folate pool before inhibition of growth occurs. Resistance emerges readily, and bacteria resistant to one sulphonamide are cross-resistant to the others. Sensitivity tests present problems in the laboratory since results depend critically on the composition of the culture medium and the inoculum size.

The emergence of resistant strains and the appearance of safer and more potent agents have relegated the sulphonamides to a minor place in therapy. Even in their traditional role, uncomplicated urinary infection, they are now seldom used. They are still found in combination products with trimethoprim, pyrimethamine, and other diaminopyrimidines (see below).

Topical silver sulfadiazine is used in burns, but the activity probably owes as much to the silver as to the sulphonamide. In curious extension of the good fortune that attended the discovery of the sulphonamides, sulfasalazine, an agent used in ulcerative colitis and rheumatoid arthritis, probably owes its efficacy to a breakdown product, 5-aminosalicylic acid.

Most sulphonamides are well absorbed when given orally and are chiefly excreted in the urine, partly in an antibacterially inactive acetylated form. The compounds diffuse relatively well into cerebrospinal fluid and were successfully used for treating meningitis before resistance became common. Sulfadiazine is effective in eradicating *Neisseria meningitidis* from the throat, provided the strain is not sulphonamide resistant.

Less soluble sulphonamides (e.g. sulfathiazole and sulfadiazine) are prone to cause renal damage due to the deposition of crystals in the urinary collecting system. Sulfafurazole (known as sulfisoxazole in the USA), sulfadimidine (sulfamethazine), sulfasomidine (sulfisomidine), and sulfamethizole lack this side effect and are preferred in the treatment of urinary infection. Some sulphonamides are distinguished by long plasma half-lives ($T\frac{1}{2}$) and are known as long-acting sulphonamides. Sulfametopyrazine

($T\frac{1}{2} = 60$ h) and sulfadoxine ($T\frac{1}{2} = 120$ h) are excreted so slowly that they are given at weekly intervals.

Diaminopyrimidines

Diaminopyrimidines inhibit dihydrofolate reductase, the enzyme that generates tetrahydrofolate (the active form of the vitamin) from metabolically inactive dihydrofolate. Trimethoprim (Fig. 3.2), the most important antibacterial agent of this type, exhibits far greater affinity for the dihydrofolate reductase of bacteria than for the corresponding mammalian enzyme; this is the basis of the selective toxicity of the compound.

Since sulphonamides and trimethoprim act at different points in the same metabolic pathway they interact synergically: bacteria are inhibited by much lower concentrations of the combination than by either agent alone. For this reason trimethoprim and sulphonamides are often combined in therapeutic formulations, although trimethoprim alone is probably as effective and less toxic. The most commonly used combination is trimethoprim and sulfamethoxazole (co-trimoxazole), but combinations of trimethoprim with sulfadiazine (co-trimazine) and sulfamoxole (co-trifamole) are also available in some countries.

Trimethoprim is active in low concentration against many common pathogenic bacteria, although *Ps. aeruginosa* is a notable exception. Resistance is on the increase; over 30% of urinary isolates have been reported to be resistant in some series, but this is not a universal experience. The drug is rapidly absorbed from the gut and excreted almost exclusively by the kidneys with a plasma half-life of about 10 h.

The chief use for trimethoprim is in urinary tract infection. The combination with sulfamethoxazole is principally used in pneumonia caused by the fungus, *Pneumocystis carinii* (*P. jiroveci*; see p. 73). It has also been extensively used in many other clinical situations, including typhoid fever, and brucellosis. Although toxic side effects are uncommon, trimethoprim–sulphonamide combinations are prone to rare, but severe side

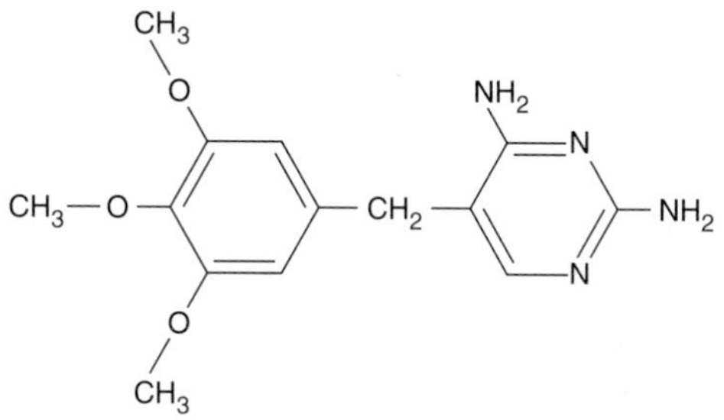

Fig. 3.2 Structure of trimethoprim.

effects (see p. 228) and it is preferable to use trimethoprim alone wherever possible.

Analogues of trimethoprim, including tetroxoprim and brodimoprim, are marketed in combination with sulphonamides in some countries, but offer few, if any advantages. Other diaminopyrimidines include the antimalarial agents pyrimethamine and proguanil (Chapter 5); the anti-pneumocystis agent trimetrexate; and the antineoplastic agent methotrexate.

Quinolones

Nalidixic acid (Fig. 3.3) was the first representative to appear of a family of compounds that share close similarities of structure. These agents are generically known as quinolones, although they embrace a variety of molecular types, depending on the arrangement of nitrogen atoms within the heterocyclic structure.

Among the earlier quinolones are two with modestly improved antibacterial activity: flumequine (which bears a fluorine atom at the C-6 position) and pipemidic acid (with a piperazine substituent at C-7). During the 1980s a new series of quinolones were synthesized in which these two features were combined. These compounds, of which ciprofloxacin (Fig. 3.3) is a typical example, exhibit considerably enhanced activity. In some subsequent derivatives, piperazine was replaced by other substituents, and members of this family of compounds are now generally referred to as fluoroquinolones. Although flumequine is strictly a fluoroquinolone, the term is usually restricted to compounds that exhibit superior intrinsic activity.

Further attempts to improve the pharmacological and antimicrobial properties of these compounds have led to the appearance of a new group of fluoroquinolones, so that these agents can now be loosely categorized into three types (Table 3.1).

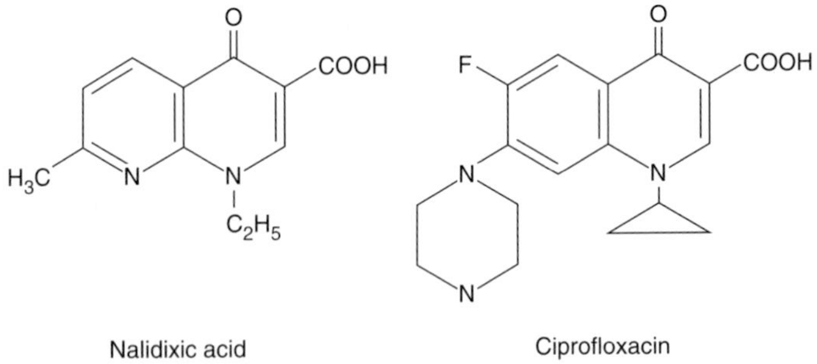

Nalidixic acid   Ciprofloxacin

Fig. 3.3 Structures of nalidixic acid and ciprofloxacin.

Table 3.1 Categorization of quinolone antibacterial agents

Narrow spectrum quinolones	Fluoroquinolones	Fluoroquinolones with improved spectrum
Acrosoxacin	Ciprofloxacin[a]	Clinafloxacin
Cinoxacin	Enoxacin	Gatifloxacin
Flumequine	Fleroxacin	Gemifloxacin
Nalidixic acid[a]	Levofloxacin[a]	Moxifloxacin[a]
Oxolinic acid	Lomefloxacin	Pazufloxacin
Pipemidic acid	Norfloxacin[a]	Sparfloxacin
Piromidic acid	Ofloxacin[a]	Tosufloxacin
	Pefloxacin	Trovafloxacin
	Rufloxacin	

[a]Compounds on the market in the UK (2006).

All antibacterial quinolones act against the remarkable enzymes that are involved in maintaining the integrity of the supercoiled DNA helix during replication and transcription. Two enzymes are affected, DNA gyrase and topoisomerase IV, so that these drugs have a dual site of action. In Gram-negative bacilli the main target is DNA gyrase, with topoisomerase IV as a secondary site, but in *Staphylococcus aureus* and some other Gram-positive cocci, the situation is reversed. Relative affinity for the two sites has led to claims of differential activity, especially among some of the newer quinolone derivatives.

Quinolones are generally well tolerated, but rashes and gastrointestinal disturbances may occur; photophobia and various non-specific neurological complaints are also sometimes encountered. These compounds affect the deposition of cartilage in experimental animals, and licensing authorities have cautioned against their use in children and pregnant women. Several promising fluoroquinolones have had to be withdrawn or have had their use restricted because of unexpected toxicity.

Nalidixic acid and its early congeners   **Uncomplicated cystitis only**

Several quinolone derivatives, including cinoxacin, oxolinic acid, and pipemidic acid, were introduced into clinical use in various countries following the marketing of nalidixic acid in the 1960s (Table 3.1, left-hand column). They are all well absorbed when taken by mouth and are more or less extensively metabolized in the body before being excreted into the urine. Nalidixic acid itself is largely converted to hydroxynalidixic acid (which retains antibacterial activity) and glucuronide conjugates (which do not).

Most Gram-negative bacteria, with the exception of *Ps. aeruginosa*, are susceptible to nalidixic acid and its early congeners, but Gram-positive organisms are usually resistant (Table 3.2). Susceptible bacteria readily develop resistance in the laboratory and the emergence of resistance sometimes occurs during treatment. These drugs are best suited to the undemanding role of the treatment of cystitis, though they are also used in gastrointestinal disease in some parts of the world. Acrosoxacin exhibits good activity against *Neisseria* and has been used for the treatment of gonorrhoea. These older quinolones offer few benefits and only nalidixic acid remains widely available.

Fluoroquinolones

After the appearance, over a 20-year period, of a series of compounds that offered little improvement over nalidixic acid, the discovery of a family of quinolones that exhibited greatly improved properties came as a surprise. These compounds, listed in the central column of Table 3.1, are much more active than earlier derivatives against enterobacteria, *Ps. aeruginosa*, and many Gram-positive cocci (Table 3.2), though the activity is somewhat reduced in acidic conditions and in the presence of divalent cations such as magnesium. The spectrum also includes certain problem organisms such as chlamydiae, legionellae, and some mycobacteria. Similar compounds, including enrofloxacin, danofloxacin, and sarafloxacin, have been introduced into veterinary practice and there has been considerable debate about the impact this may have had on the development of resistance.

The success of the first fluoroquinolones led to an intensive search for derivatives with further improved properties and this has borne fruit with several new agents now on the world market, or at an advanced stage of development (Table 3.1, right-hand column). These compounds are characterized by enhanced activity against Gram-positive cocci, including *Staph. aureus* and *Streptococcus pneumoniae* as well as chlamydiae and mycoplasmas; clinafloxacin, gatifloxacin, moxifloxacin, and trovafloxacin also have sufficient activity against anaerobes of the *Bacteroides fragilis* group to make treatment of infections with those organisms feasible. They are not reliably active against *Ps. aeruginosa*.

Fluoroquinolones are usually administered orally, although some, including ciprofloxacin, ofloxacin, levofloxacin (the L-isomer of ofloxacin), and trovafloxacin (in the form of its pro-drug, alatrofloxacin), can also be given

Table 3.2 Summary of spectrum of activity of quinolones available in the UK (2006)

Quinolone	Enterobacteria	*Pseudomonas aeruginosa*	Staphylococci	Streptococci	*Bacteroides fragilis*	Chlamydiae
Ciprofloxacin	Very good	Good	Good	Fair	Poor	Poor
Levofloxacin	Very good	Good	Good	Fair	Fair	Good
Moxifloxacin	Very good	Poor	Very good	Good	Fair	Good
Nalidixic acid	Good	Poor	Poor	Poor	Poor	Poor
Norfloxacin	Very good	Good	Fair	Poor	Poor	Poor
Ofloxacin	Very good	Good	Fair	Fair	Poor	Fair

by injection. Therapeutic dosages achieve relatively low concentrations in plasma, but the compounds are well distributed in tissues and are concentrated within mammalian cells. The major route of excretion is usually renal, in the form of native compound or glucuronide and other metabolites, some of which retain antibacterial activity. Some fluoroquinolones, notably rufloxacin and sparfloxacin, but also including moxifloxacin, and trovafloxacin, exhibit long terminal half-lives; these compounds are partly excreted by the biliary route and this may help to explain the long half-life.

Among currently available fluoroquinolones, norfloxacin, enoxacin, and lomefloxacin have found their greatest use as more reliable replacements for earlier derivatives in the treatment of urinary tract infection, though they may also have wider uses, for example in gonococcal and gastrointestinal infections. Others are used for systemic infection and have become the subject of conflicting marketing claims. Ciprofloxacin is the most widely used; among other indications, it is now the drug of choice for typhoid fever and other serious enteric diseases. The ease of administration of fluoroquinolones makes them attractive candidates for 'blind' therapy in hospital and domiciliary practice. However, they are not universal panaceas and should not be used indiscriminately. The newer derivatives are being targeted at the treatment of respiratory infections in the community and, although they are undoubtedly effective, it is not clear that such use is necessary or wise. Indeed, there is already evidence that indiscriminate use of fluoroquinolones is undermining the effectiveness of these valuable drugs by encouraging resistance, notably in Gram-negative bacilli and pneumococci.

Nitroimidazoles   **Anaerobic infections only**

As a group, the imidazoles are remarkable in that derivatives are known, which between them cover bacteria, fungi, viruses, protozoa, and helminths—in fact, the whole antimicrobial spectrum. Outside the antimicrobial field certain imidazoles have been shown to exhibit radio-sensitizing properties and have attracted attention as adjuncts to radiation therapy for some tumours.

The members of this family of compounds used as antibacterial agents are 5-nitroimidazoles, of which metronidazole (Fig. 3.4) is best known. Related 5-nitroimidazoles include tinidazole, ornidazole, secnidazole, and nimorazole; they share the properties of metronidazole but have longer plasma half-lives.

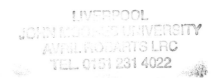

Fig. 3.4 Structure of metronidazole.

Metronidazole was originally used for the treatment of trichomoniasis, and subsequently for two other protozoal infections—amoebiasis and giardiasis. The antibacterial activity of the compound was first recognized when a patient suffering from acute ulcerative gingivitis responded spontaneously while receiving metronidazole for a *Trichomonas vaginalis* infection. Anaerobic bacteria are commonly incriminated in gingivitis, and it was subsequently shown that metronidazole possesses potent antibacterial activity that was originally thought to be confined to strict anaerobes (the protozoa against which the drug is effective also exhibit anaerobic metabolism) since even oxygen-tolerant species such as *Actinomyces* and *Propionibacterium* are resistant. However, some micro-aerophilic bacteria, including *Gardnerella vaginalis* and *Helicobacter pylori*, are commonly susceptible to nitroimidazoles, and metronidazole features in drug regimens for the treatment of infections with these organisms.

Metronidazole is so effective against anaerobic bacteria and resistance is so uncommon that it is now the drug of choice for the treatment of anaerobic infections. It is also commonly used for prophylaxis in some surgical procedures in which postoperative anaerobic infection is a frequent complication. It is the preferred alternative to vancomycin in the treatment of antibiotic-associated colitis caused by *Clostridium difficile* toxins (p. 303).

The basis of the selective activity against anaerobes resides in the fact that a reduction product is produced intracellularly at the low redox values attainable by anaerobes, but not by aerobes. The reduced form of metronidazole is thought to induce strand breakage in DNA by a mechanism that has not been precisely determined.

The 5-nitroimidazoles are generally free from serious side effects, though gastrointestinal upset is common and ingestion of alcohol induces a disulfiram-like reaction. Since these drugs act on DNA they are potentially genotoxic and tumorigenic, but there is no evidence that these problems have arisen despite widespread clinical use. None the less, these compounds are best avoided in pregnancy.

Nitrofurans   Urinary tract infection only (nitrofurantoin)

A number of nitrofuran derivatives have attracted attention over the years, among which nitrofurantoin (Fig. 3.5) is much the most important. Others include furazolidone (an orally compound sometimes used for intestinal infections); nitrofurazone (a topical agent also used for bladder irrigation); nifuratel and nifuroxime (used in some countries for *T. vaginalis* infection and vaginal thrush); and nifurtimox (used in Chagas' disease; see p. 429).

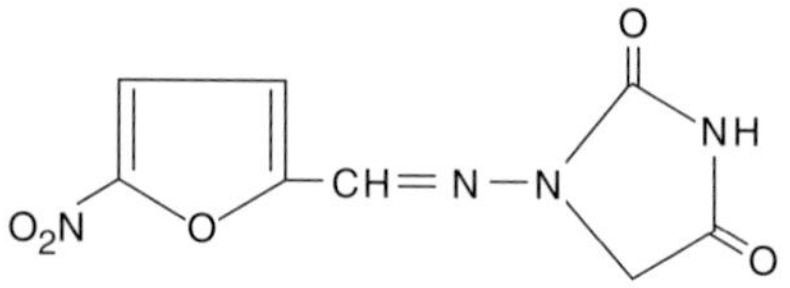

Fig. 3.5 Structure of nitrofurantoin.

Nitrofurantoin is the only nitrofuran derivative available in the UK. Its use is restricted to the treatment of urinary infection since it is rapidly excreted into urine after oral absorption and the small amount that finds its way into tissues is inactivated there. It is active against most urinary tract pathogens, but *Proteus* spp. and *Ps. aeruginosa* are usually resistant. The occurrence of resistant strains among susceptible species is uncommon. The activity is affected by pH, being favoured by acid conditions.

Nausea is fairly common after administration of nitrofurantoin; macro-crystalline formulations have improved gastrointestinal tolerance and are generally preferred for this reason.

The mode of action of nitrofurantoin (or other nitrofurans) has not been precisely elucidated and is probably complex. The nitro group is reduced intracellularly in susceptible bacteria and it is likely that one effect, as with metronidazole, is the interaction of a reduction product with DNA.

Rifamycins   Mainly mycobacterial infections

The clinically useful rifamycins, of which rifampicin (known in the USA as rifampin) is the most important, are semisynthetic derivatives of rifamycin B, one of a group of structurally complex antibiotics produced by *Streptomyces mediterranei*. These compounds interfere with mRNA formation by binding to the β-subunit of DNA-dependent RNA polymerase. Resistance readily arises by mutations in the subunit. For this reason, the drugs are normally used in combination with other agents.

Rifampicin

Rifampicin is one of the most effective weapons against two major mycobacterial scourges of mankind: tuberculosis and leprosy. It also exhibits potent bactericidal activity against a range of other bacteria, notably staphylococci and legionellae. Rifampicin is such a useful antimycobacterial drug that there has been a move to confine its use to tuberculosis and leprosy on the grounds that more widespread use might inadvertently encourage the emergence of resistant strains of mycobacteria. Critics of this view claim that an agent that possesses exceptionally good antistaphylococcal activity and useful activity against other bacteria is being unnecessarily restricted on unproven grounds. In fact, restriction of the use of rifampicin has been steadily eroded: it is now often used in combination with erythromycin in Legionnaires' disease; it is also used to eliminate meningococci from the throats of carriers and for the protection of close contacts of meningococcal and *Haemophilus influenzae* type b disease.

Rifampicin is well absorbed by the oral route, although it may also be given by intravenous infusion. Serious side effects are relatively uncommon, but can be more troublesome when the drug is used intermittently, as it may be in antituberculosis regimens. Hepatotoxicity is well recognized and the antibiotic induces hepatic enzymes, leading to self-potentiation of excretion and antagonism of some other drugs handled by the liver, including oral contraceptives. A potentially alarming side effect arising from the fact that rifampicin is strongly pigmented is the production of red urine and other bodily secretions; contact lenses may become discoloured. Patients should be warned of these potential problems.

Other rifamycins

Two other rifamycin derivatives are of particular interest: rifapentine exhibits an extended plasma half-life, but is otherwise similar to rifampicin; rifabutin (ansamycin) also has a prolonged half-life and retains activity against some rifampicin-resistant bacteria. Much interest has focused on the possibility that these agents may be useful in infections caused by organisms of the *Mycobacterium avium* complex, which often cause disseminated disease in patients with cancer or acquired immune deficiency syndrome (AIDS). Although these mycobacteria are commonly resistant to standard anti-tuberculosis drugs, rifabutin and rifapentine display good activity in vitro. Clinical success has been modest, but rifabutin has proved of sufficient value to warrant its inclusion in some multidrug regimens for prophylaxis against infection with organisms of the *M. avium* complex.

Rifaximin, rifamide, and rifamycin SV are poorly absorbed after oral administration. Although they are marketed in some countries for gastrointestinal infections and for topical application, they are not recommended.

Agents affecting membrane function

Polymyxins   Pseudomonas infections only

The polymyxins are a family of compounds produced by *Bacillus polymyxa* and related bacteria. Only polymyxins B and E are used therapeutically. Polymyxin E is usually known by its alternative name, colistin. Structurally, the polymyxins are cyclic polypeptides with a long hydrophobic tail. They act like cationic detergents by binding to the cell membrane and causing the leakage of essential cytoplasmic contents. The effect is not entirely selective, and both polymyxin B and colistin exhibit considerable toxicity.

Derivatives of the polymyxins in which up to five diaminobutyric acid residues are substituted with sulphomethyl groups are better tolerated and more quickly excreted than the parent compounds. These sulphomethyl polymyxins exhibit diminished antibacterial activity, but the precise loss in activity is difficult to estimate because the substituted compounds spontaneously break down to the more active parent.

The antibacterial spectrum of the polymyxins encompasses most Gram-negative bacteria except *Proteus* spp., but the importance of these antibiotics hinges on their activity against *Ps. aeruginosa*. With the appearance of antipseudomonal β-lactam agents, aminoglycosides, and fluoroquinolones, the polymyxins have virtually fallen into disuse for systemic therapy, although they are still used in some topical preparations. They are also included in selective decontamination regimens aimed at preventing endogenous infection in profoundly neutropenic patients (p. 403) and there are advocates of the use of colistin in cystic fibrosis by instillation into the lungs of those suffering exacerbation of pseudomonal infection.

Other membrane-active agents

Daptomycin, a semi-synthetic lipopeptide antibiotic not unlike the polymyxins in structure, has various effects on bacteria, but the primary mode of action is thought to lie in disruption of the cell membrane. Development of the compound in the 1980s was stopped because of fears of toxicity, but the rise to prominence of multiresistant Gram-positive cocci revived commercial interest and it is now marketed for serious infections of the skin and soft tissues that are unresponsive to other agents, especially those caused by multiresistant staphylococci. Activity is restricted to Gram-positive cocci and is greatly enhanced in vitro by the presence of magnesium ions.

Antibiotics of the tyrothricin complex (gramicidin and tyrocidine), which are used in some topical preparations, are cyclic peptides that bind to the cell membrane and interfere with its function. These agents possess good activity against Gram-positive organisms, but they also bind to mammalian cell membranes and are far too toxic to be used systemically in humans.

Toxicity also precludes the systemic use of the many disinfectants, including phenols, quaternary ammonium compounds, biguanides, and others, that achieve their antibacterial effect wholly or in part by interfering with the integrity of the cell membrane.

Naturally occurring oligopeptides that destabilize bacterial membranes are widespread in nature, where they play a part in innate defence against microbial infection. Compounds of this type include cecropins (originally described in insects), magainins (from frogs), defensins (from mammalian leucocytes), and lanthionine-containing 'lantibiotics' (from bacteria). Whether these, or related synthetic compounds, have any future as therapeutic agents remains to be seen.

Antimycobacterial agents

Compared with the number of agents at the disposal of the prescriber for the therapy of most bacterial infections, the resources available to treat mycobacterial disease are precariously meagre. Part of the reason is that mycobacteria are unusual organisms with a relatively impermeable waxy coat, but the fact that they are very slow growing and are able to survive and multiply within macrophages and necrotic tissue also makes them difficult targets.

In general, the development of drugs for the treatment of tuberculosis and leprosy has evolved along specialized lines, but some important antimycobacterial agents, such as rifampicin (see above) and certain aminoglycosides (Chapter 2), have wider uses. Agents specifically used for the treatment of tuberculosis include isoniazid (isonicotinic acid hydrazide), pyrazinamide, ethambutol, and thiacetazone (thioacetazone). *Para*-aminosalicylic acid, which was formerly much used in antituberculosis regimens, is no longer recommended, but this and other compounds with activity against *Mycobacterium tuberculosis*, such as capreomycin, cycloserine, and viomycin, may be considered if first-line treatment fails. In leprosy, the most important agents (apart from rifampicin) are dapsone (or its pro-drug, acedapsone) and clofazimine. The thioamides ethionamide and protionamide (prothionamide) are sometimes used, but are hepatotoxic.

Some fluoroquinolones and macrolides display quite good activity against mycobacteria, including *M. leprae* and organisms of the *M. avium* complex, and these agents widen the options for treating mycobacterial disease at a time when resistance is emerging as a serious problem.

Because of the difficulties in studying mycobacteria in the laboratory, less is known about the mode of action of antimycobacterial drugs than about other antibacterial agents. Various theories have been put forward to explain the action of isoniazid. The most widely held view is that an oxidized product inhibits the formation of the mycolic acids that are peculiar to the cell walls of acid-fast bacilli. Other derivatives of nicotinic acid, including pyrazinamide, ethionamide, and protionamide, may act in the same way. Ethambutol probably inhibits the formation of arabinogalactan, a polysaccharide component of the mycobacterial cell wall. Dapsone (diaminodiphenyl sulphone) and *para*-aminosalicylic acid are related to the sulphonamides and have been assumed to share the same mode of action, but this is by no means certain. The mode of action of the antileprosy agent clofazimine has not been determined, but it may, like rifampicin, inhibit DNA-dependent RNA polymerase. Some puzzling aspects of the idiosyncratic spectrum of antimycobacterial agents may be explained by differences in uptake into susceptible cells.

Further information on these agents is given in the context of their use in Chapter 25.

Miscellaneous antibacterial agents: prescriber's survival kit

- *Trimethoprim*: use alone for uncomplicated cystitis
- *Ciprofloxacin*: good general purpose fluoroquinolone. Do not use in pneumococcal pneumonia
- *Norfloxacin*: useful for uncomplicated cystitis
- *Metronidazole*: drug of choice for anaerobic infections
- *Rifampicin*: essential component of regimens for treatment of tuberculosis and leprosy

Chapter 4

Antifungal agents

Fungi may cause benign but unsightly infection of the skin, nail, or hair (dermatophytosis), relatively trivial infection of mucous membranes (thrush), or systemic infection causing progressive, often fatal disease. The taxonomy of fungi is highly complex, but for medical purposes they are commonly considered in four morphological groups:

- yeasts that reproduce by budding (e.g. *Cryptococcus neoformans*)
- yeasts that produce a pseudomycelium (e.g. *Candida albicans*)
- filamentous fungi (moulds) that produce a true mycelium (e.g. *Aspergillus fumigatus*)
- dimorphic fungi that grow as yeasts or filamentous fungi, depending on the cultural conditions (e.g. *Histoplasma capsulatum*).

In addition, *Pneumocystis carinii*, an important opportunist pathogen, especially of patients with AIDS, is now regarded as a fungus. The nomenclature is in dispute and the organism is sometimes referred to as *Pneumocystis jiroveci*.

Fungi are eukaryotic organisms and antibacterial agents are generally ineffective against them. Specialized antifungal agents must therefore be used, and some are quite toxic. In order to minimize problems of toxicity, superficial lesions are usually treated by topical application, but deep mycoses, which are serious life-threatening infections, need vigorous systemic therapy. Unfortunately, therapeutic resources for the treatment of systemic mycoses are slender. The polyene amphotericin B is the mainstay; otherwise choice is limited to flucytosine, a handful of azole derivatives (mainly triazoles), and a new group of semisynthetic antibiotics, the echinocandins. *P. carinii* is insusceptible to conventional antifungal agents, and alternative treatment regimens have been devised.

The differential activity of the main antifungal agents in common use is summarized in Table 4.1. Precise assessment of the activity of antifungal agents in vitro is beset with methodological difficulties and susceptibility tests are not generally available, except in reference centres.

Table 4.1 Summary of the differential activity of antifungal agents against the more common pathogenic fungi

Fungus	Principal diseases caused	Polyenes	Flucytosine	Griseofulvin	Azoles	Allylamines	Echinocandins
Yeasts							
Cryptococcus neoformans	Meningitis	+	+	-	+	-	-
Candida albicans	Thrush; systemic candidiasis	+	+	-	+	±	+
Filamentous fungi							
Trichophyton spp.	Infection of skin, nail or hair ('ringworm')	-	+	+	+	-	
Microsporum spp.						-	
Epidermophyton floccosum						-	
Aspergillus fumigatus	Pulmonary aspergillosis	+	-	-	(+)^a	(+)^b	+
Dimorphic fungi							
Histoplasma capsulatum	Histoplasmosis	+			+		-
Coccidioides immitis	Coccidioidomycosis		-	-	+	(+)^b	-
Blastomyces dermatitidis	Blastomycosis						-

+, useful activity; −, no useful activity.

[a] Variable activity; itraconazole and voriconazole are most active.

[b] Clinical efficacy not yet established.

especially when administered in a liposomal formulation that carries the drug into macrophages. The antifungal azoles (p. 70), the aminoglycoside, paromomycin, and pentamidine also exhibit some activity against leishmania and offer alternatives in recalcitrant cases. Much hope for leishmaniasis sufferers rests with an oral phosphocholine analogue, miltefosine, which has undergone successful trials in visceral leishmaniasis in India and also shows signs of benefit in cutaneous forms of the disease.

Other flagellates

Two other flagellates cause disease in man: *Giardia lamblia* (also known as *G. intestinalis*)—a common cause of diarrhoea, abdominal pain, and steatorrhoea—and *Trichomonas vaginalis*, a common cause of vaginitis or, more rarely, urethritis. *G. lamblia* is transmitted in the cyst form, often in infected water; *T. vaginalis* is transmitted venereally. Both of these parasites are susceptible to nitroimidazoles such as metronidazole (p. 60). Resistance is uncommon. Mepacrine (known in the USA as quinacrine), and the anthelminthic benzimidazole albendazole also exhibit effective antigiardial activity, but there are few alternatives for refractory trichomoniasis—except, perhaps, polyenes such as natamycin and trichomycin (p. 69), which are available in some countries.

Sporozoa

The sporozoa are all parasitic; they have a complex life cycle involving alternate sexual and asexual phases. Among important human parasites are the malaria parasites and the coccidia.

Malaria parasites

Malaria is the most important of all parasitic diseases. It remains the commonest cause of fever in the world and is a major cause of morbidity and mortality in areas of high endemicity throughout the tropical belt. Four species infect man. *Plasmodium falciparum* is the most dangerous, since primary infections are often rapidly fatal if left untreated. *P. vivax* and *P. ovale*, which cause benign tertian malaria, and *P. malariae*, which causes quartan malaria, rarely kill but give rise to debilitating infections. The most common species worldwide is *P. falciparum*, which accounts for over 90% of infections in tropical Africa; in some parts of the world, notably the Indian subcontinent, *P. vivax* is the dominant species.

The malaria parasite is transmitted by the bite of infected female *Anopheles* mosquitoes. The parasites first infect liver cells; then after 1–2 weeks the liver parasites mature and infect circulating red blood cells to commence the cycle of erythrocytic schizogony, which is responsible for the overt signs of disease. *P. vivax* and *P. ovale* can also set up a cryptic infection in the liver, which may cause the relapse of symptoms up to 2 years after the infection is acquired. A proportion of erythrocytic parasites differentiate into male and female gametocytes, which do not develop further in the mammalian host but complete the sexual phase of development in the anopheline vector when ingested during a blood meal.

The traditional mainstay of the treatment of malaria is quinine, the active principle of the bark of the cinchona tree brought to Europe from South America in the seventeenth century, but various other effective antimalarials have been developed. These include the 4-aminoquinolines chloroquine and amodiaquine, which act on erythrocytic parasites, and the 8-aminoquinolines primaquine, bulaquine (a primaquine analogue available in India) and tafenoquine (an investigational compound with an extended half-life), which are selectively active against the liver forms. Quinine and the 4-aminoquinolines are thought to achieve their effect by preventing the polymerization of haem (ferriprotoporphyrin IX), a reaction that is needed to detoxify this product of parasite metabolism within red blood cells. Primaquine appears to act in a different way, possibly by interfering with mitochondrial enzymes.

A group of compounds collectively known as 'antifolates' are also used, usually in combination, especially for antimalarial prophylaxis. These include pyrimethamine, proguanil, (and chlorproguanil) the long-acting sulphonamides, sulfadoxine and sulfalene (sulfametopyrazine), and dapsone (p. 65). Pyrimethamine, a dihydrofolate reductase inhibitor related to trimethoprim (p. 55), exhibits a selectively high affinity for the plasmodial form of the enzyme and interacts synergically with sulphonamides. Proguanil and chlorproguanil are biguanides that are metabolized in the body to compounds closely related to pyrimethamine, and have an identical mode of action. Surprisingly, some pyrimethamine-resistant mutants retain susceptibility to these closely related compounds. Chlorproguanil (Lapudrine) combined with dapsone—'lapdap'—is being promoted in parts of Africa as a relatively cheap treatment for malaria with a reduced propensity to generate resistance. Proguanil itself is used solely for prophylaxis, usually together with chloroquine. A combination with atovaquone (a hydroxynaphthoquinone that acts on the respiratory chain of some protozoa) is available for treatment and prophylaxis.

Resistance to chloroquine and most other antimalarial agents is now common in *P. falciparum* in many parts of the world. Quinine remains reliably active against most strains, and this old compound is still widely used for the treatment of falciparum malaria, but derivatives of artemisinin, the active principle of an ancient Chinese herbal remedy, qinghaosu, are more rapidly effective and are gaining acceptance. Formulations include the water-soluble artesunate, and the oily solutions, artemether, and artemotil (β-arteether) all of which are suitable for intramuscular injection. Artesunate can also be given intravenously and by mouth. Some formulations, including artemisinin itself, can be administered rectally. Certain antibiotics, notably tetracyclines and clindamycin, have antimalarial activity and are used as adjuncts to artemisinin or quinine therapy in chloroquine-resistant falciparum malaria. Chloroquine-resistant strains usually remain susceptible to mefloquine and halofantrine, quinoline derivatives developed by the Walter Reed Army Institute of Research in Washington, but resistance to these agents is also beginning to appear. Lumefantrine (formerly known as benflumetol), appears to lack the cardiotoxicity of halofantrine and is now generally preferred, but it is available only as an oral combination product with artemether.

Coccidia

Phylogenetically related to the malaria parasites are the coccidia, which share many features of the complex life cycle, but are not transmitted by insect vectors. Several species, including *Cryptosporidium parvum*, *Isospora belli*, and *Cyclospora cayetanensis* cause diarrhoea in man. Infection is usually self-limiting, but in immunocompromised patients, especially those suffering from AIDS, they may cause severe and protracted symptoms. Nitazoxanide, a nitrothiazole derivative, which is converted in the body to the active form, tizoxanide, seems to offer effective therapy against *C. parvum* if antimicrobial treatment is necessary. Infections with *I. belli* and *Cyclo. cayetanensis* respond to co-trimoxazole, though antimicrobial therapy is seldom required.

The most important human coccidian parasite is *Toxoplasma gondii*. Intrauterine infections with this organism are an important cause of congenital malformations and stillbirth throughout the world. AIDS sufferers may develop toxoplasma encephalitis, apparently by reactivation of latent infection. Cats often harbour the parasite and liberate the infectious oocysts in their faeces; this probably represents a major reservoir of infection, although undercooked meat is also a recognized source. Pyrimethamine, in combination with a sulphonamide (usually sulfadiazine) is the treatment of choice in toxoplasmosis. Clindamycin and the macrolide antibiotic spiramycin have also been successfully used, especially in combination with pyrimethamine. Spiramycin has been recommended during pregnancy, when antifolates are best avoided.

Other protozoa

Babesia spp., like malaria parasites, infect red blood cells, but they are unrelated. They are predominantly animal parasites that are occasionally transmitted to man by the bite of ixodid ticks. Recorded European cases have mostly been in splenectomized patients and have usually been caused by *B. divergens*. Infection with *B. microti* occurs in previously healthy persons in parts of North America.

Balantidium coli is a ciliate, cosmopolitan in distribution, which is a rare cause of severe diarrhoea. *Encephalitozoon cuniculi* and some other microsporidia occasionally cause infection, usually in immunocompromised patients. Although these protozoa have ribosomes of the prokaryotic type, inhibitors of bacterial protein synthesis do not seem to work.

Treatment of babesiosis and infection with assorted intestinal protozoa is generally ill-defined. Options for therapy are considered in Chapter 30.

Antiprotozoal drugs: prescriber's survival kit

- *Quinine*: emergency treatment for suspected falciparum malaria
- *Chloroquine*: treatment of vivax, ovale and quartan malaria
- *Primaquine*: prevention of relapse; vivax and ovale malaria
- *Metronidazole*: first choice for trichomoniasis, giardiasis, amoebiasis
- *All other protozoal infections*: leave to the experts

Helminths

Helminths are parasitic worms. They often have a complex life cycle involving a period of development outside the definitive host either in soil or in an intermediate host. Helminths of medical importance fall into three major groups: nematodes (roundworms), trematodes (flukes), and cestodes (tapeworms) (Table 5.2).

Little work is done on the development of anthelminthic agents for use in human beings, and most agents in present use have emerged through application of drugs originally intended for the treatment of animals. Despite this, a wide variety of compounds is available for use in worm infections and, astonishingly, there are now three compounds—ivermectin, praziquantel, and albendazole—which between them cover virtually the whole helminthic spectrum. Resistance to these agents is known to occur in animals, and there

Chapter 6

Antiviral agents

Viruses are almost as versatile as bacteria in the range of diseases they can cause. Vertebrates, insects, plants, and even bacteria are all open to attack. Some viruses of vertebrates (arboviruses) develop in and are transmitted by mosquitoes or other arthropods; others—rabies is a good example—can infect a wide range of mammalian hosts. In general, however, viruses are highly specific in their host range.

All viruses are obligate intracellular parasites; that is, they replicate only within living cells and cannot usually survive for long outside the host cell. Selectivity usually extends not only to the host, but also to the type of cell within the host, as viruses only infect cells that express appropriate receptors on their surface. The preference of a virus for certain types of cell is known as the tropism of the virus, and this often accounts for the characteristic clinical manifestations of particular viral infections. Thus, some viruses preferentially infect liver cells, giving rise to hepatitis.

Most viruses that infect man gain entry to the body by adsorption to superficial cells of the mucous membranes of the respiratory, intestinal, and genital tracts, or of the conjunctivae. Others find their way in through damaged skin, insect bites, or direct inoculation. Intact skin is normally impermeable to viruses, although wart virus is an exception.

The principal types of virus causing human disease are listed in Table 6.1.

Properties of viruses

Viruses are deceptively simple. Sizes range from about 20 nm (parvovirus) to 300 nm (poxvirus); consequently, even the biggest viruses fall barely within the limits of resolution of conventional light microscopy and the electron microscope must be used to visualize them.

Complete virus particles (virions) consist of a nucleic acid core (the viral genome), surrounded by a few proteins, and possibly a lipid envelope. The nucleic acid may be DNA or RNA (never both), single or double stranded, circular or linear, continuous or segmented. This provides all the information needed for viral replication once it is released within the host cell. The proteins serve a number of functions. The capsid, or protein coat surrounding

Table 6.1 Principal types of virus causing human disease

Family	Examples	Diseases	Mode of transmission
RNA Viruses			
Orthomyxoviruses	Influenza A and B viruses	Influenza	Respiratory
Paramyxoviruses	Mumps virus	Mumps	Respiratory
	Measles virus	Measles	Respiratory
	Respiratory syncytial virus	Bronchiolitis (especially babies)	Respiratory
	Human metapneumovirus	Bronchiolitis (especially babies)	Respiratory
	Parainfluenza viruses	Croup; bronchiolitis (especially babies)	Respiratory
Rhabdoviruses	Rabies virus	Rabies	Bite of rabid animal
Arenaviruses	Lassa virus	Lassa fever	Respiratory/rodent reservoir
Togaviruses	Rubella virus	German measles (rubella)	Respiratory/congenital
Flaviviruses	Many arboviruses	Yellow fever	Arthropod vectors
	Hepatitis C virus	Hepatitis	Inoculation

Group	Virus	Disease	Transmission
Picornaviruses	Enteroviruses:	Polio; meningitis; paralysis	Faecal–oral
	Echo	Meningitis	
	Coxsackie A and B	Meningitis	
	Hepatitis A virus	Infectious hepatitis	
	Rhinoviruses	Colds	Respiratory
Retroviruses	Human immunodeficiency viruses	AIDS	Inoculation/sexual/vertical
	Human T-cell lymphotropic viruses	T-cell leukaemia; lymphoma	Inoculation/sexual/vertical
Reoviruses	Rotavirus	Infantile diarrhoea	Faecal–oral
Caliciviruses	Norovirus (Norwalk virus)	Gastroenteritis	Faecal–oral
Coronaviruses	Human coronavirus	Severe acute respiratory syndrome (SARS)	Respiratory

Table 6.1 (continued) Principal types of virus causing human disease

Family	Examples	Diseases	Mode of transmission
DNA Viruses			
Poxviruses	Variola	Smallpox (now eradicated)	Mainly respiratory
	Vaccinia	Smallpox vaccine	Vaccination
	Molluscum contagiosum	Skin disease	Contact
	Orf	Skin disease	Contact with sheep
Herpesviruses	Herpes simplex virus types 1 and 2	Cold sores; genital herpes	Saliva/contact/sexual
	Varicella zoster	Chickenpox; shingles	Respiratory
	Cytomegalovirus	Non-specific illness	Close contact/kissing
	Epstein–Barr virus	Glandular fever	Saliva, e.g. kissing
	Human herpesvirus type 6	Roseola infantum (sixth disease)	Saliva
	Human herpesvirus type 7	Not known	Saliva
	Human herpesvirus type 8	Kaposi's sarcoma	Sexual
Adenoviruses	Many serotypes	Conjunctivitis; pharyngitis; infantile diarrhoea	Respiratory
Papovaviruses	Papillomaviruses	Cervical cancer; Warts	Contact
Hepadnaviruses	Hepatitis B virus	Serum hepatitis	Inoculation/sexual/vertical
Parvoviruses	Parvovirus B19	Erythema infectiosum (fifth disease)	Respiratory

or suppression of antibody production, stimulation of T-cell activity, and stimulation of expression of HLA class I and II molecules on the surface of cells. Finally, IFNs affect cell proliferation, which has led to their successful use in the management of certain malignant tumours.

When IFNs were discovered, they were hailed as the antiviral equivalent of penicillin. As these substances were produced by cells as a natural defence in response to a wide range of virus infections, it seemed reasonable to imagine that when used as therapeutic agents, they would exhibit a broad antiviral spectrum, and that their toxic effects on host cells would be minimal. Early studies were hampered by difficulties in obtaining sufficient quantities of IFNs to conduct clinical trials. This problem has been solved by recombinant DNA technology, which has allowed cloning and expression of the relevant genes, and by the use of Sendai virus to induce IFN production by a lymphoblastoid cell line (so-called lymphoblastoid IFN). Unexpectedly, clinical trials revealed that patients receiving IFN experienced flu-like side effects: fever, headache, and myalgia. This led to the realization that individuals suffering from influenza complain of flu-like symptoms precisely because of the induction of IFNs by the virus. Most patients become tolerant to these effects after the first few doses.

IFN-α is successfully used in the management of patients with chronic viral hepatitis, but the therapeutic effect may be due to its immunomodulatory rather than antiviral properties. A formulation in which a polyethylene glycol unit has been linked to IFN-α (peginterferon) has an extended half-life, is better tolerated and, most importantly, produces a much superior virological response.

Prevention of virus infections

Prevention rather than cure plays such an important part in the control of viral diseases that an appreciation of the methods used is essential to understanding the complementary role of antiviral agents. The scourge of smallpox has been removed by appropriate use of vaccinia vaccine and certain other viral infections may be similarly eradicated. The World Health Organization campaign to eliminate polio is progressing towards a successful conclusion, and in many developed countries measles, mumps, and rubella are becoming rare.

Passive immunization

Immune globulin

The transfer of preformed antibodies from one individual to another can be achieved with human gammaglobulin derived from the blood of healthy individuals known to have high antibody titres. In the days before an effective vaccine against hepatitis A became available, normal human immunoglobulin obtained from pooled routine blood donations was widely used for the protection of individuals visiting countries where the virus is common. Other types of immunoglobulin are obtained specifically from known hyperimmune individuals. Those in current use include immunoglobulin preparations against: hepatitis B, varicella zoster, rabies, vaccinia, and tetanus.

Monoclonal antibody

Techniques allowing the production of monoclonal antibodies with their exceptional intrinsic specificity have led to investigation of such compounds in the prevention of viral infection. The only one presently available, palivizumab, is a monoclonal antibody directed against respiratory syncytial virus. It is administered by intramuscular injection to vulnerable infants at monthly intervals during the autumn and winter—seasons of greatest risk of infection with the virus.

Active immunization

The host can be stimulated to produce a protective immune response by vaccination with a form of the infectious agent that does not cause disease. Vaccines can be alive or dead. Live vaccines consist of attenuated forms of the infectious agent. Examples include measles, mumps, rubella, and live poliovirus (Sabin) vaccines.

Dead vaccines may consist of the whole agent, grown in the laboratory and subsequently killed by some means, or of a subunit of the agent, usually prepared by recombinant DNA technology. Dead vaccines have the advantage that there is no risk of reversion to virulence. However, they are less immunogenic than live vaccines, and therefore more doses need to be given to achieve a satisfactory response. Examples of such vaccines include the Salk polio vaccine (now generally preferred to the live Sabin vaccine), rabies virus, hepatitis A and hepatitis B virus vaccines; the latter is a subunit vaccine, consisting only of the surface protein (HBsAg), prepared by cloning and expressing the appropriate gene in yeast cells.

Part 2

Resistance to antimicrobial agents

Chapter 8

The problem of resistance

What is resistance?

Bacterial isolates have been categorized as being susceptible or resistant to antibiotics ever since they became available. Some of the criteria on which this categorization has been based are discussed in Chapter 12, where the concepts of the minimum inhibitory concentrations (MIC) and minimum bactericidal concentrations of an antibiotic are described. Unfortunately, making an accurate judgement about microbial susceptibility or resistance is somewhat less straightforward than this traditional working definition, since there is usually no simple relationship between the MIC (or minimum bactericidal concentrations) of an antibiotic and clinical response. Therapeutic success depends not only on the concentration of the antibiotic achieved at the site of infection (i.e. its pharmacokinetic behaviour) and its activity against the infecting organisms encountered there (i.e. its pharmacodynamic behaviour), but also on the contribution that the host's own defences are able to make towards clearance of the offending microbes.

The decision as to whether a given bacterial isolate should be labelled susceptible or resistant depends ultimately on the likelihood that an infection with that organism can be expected to respond to treatment with a given drug, but microbiologists and clinicians have become accustomed to the idea that an organism is 'resistant' when it is inhibited in vitro by an antibiotic concentration that is greater than that achievable in vivo. Importantly the concentration of antibiotic that is achievable will vary according to the site of infection, dosage, and route of administration. For example, some antibiotics, such as trimethoprim, are excreted primarily via the kidneys and therefore achieve, in the context of urinary tract infections, advantageously high concentrations in urine. Furthermore, the intrinsic activity of an antibiotic against some bacteria (e.g. staphylococci) may be greater than for others (e.g. *Escherichia coli*) because of the effect of cell envelope structure on achievable intracellular antibiotic concentrations. These issues mean that several different thresholds (breakpoint concentrations) are often used to define susceptibility to an antibiotic. For example, an *Esch. coli* strain for which the MIC of ampicillin is 32 mg/l might be classed as susceptible if isolated from a urinary infection, while the same bacterium causing a blood-stream infection would be classified as ampicillin resistant. These differences in definition of susceptibility relate to the variations in achievable concentrations at the site of infection: while an ampicillin concentration of 32 mg/l can reliably be achieved in urine, this is not the case in blood.

Intrinsic resistance

If whole bacterial species are considered, rather than individual isolates, it is apparent immediately that they are not all intrinsically susceptible to all antibiotics (Table 8.1); for example, a coliform infection would not be treated with erythromycin, or a streptococcal infection with an aminoglycoside, since the organisms are intrinsically resistant to these antibiotics. Similarly, *Pseudomonas aeruginosa* and *Mycobacterium tuberculosis* are intrinsically resistant to most of the agents used to treat more tractable infections. Such intrinsically resistant organisms are sometimes termed non-susceptible, with the term resistant reserved for variants of normally susceptible species that acquire mechanism(s) of resistance (Chapter 9).

A microbe will be intrinsically resistant to an antibiotic if it either does not possess a target for the drug's action, or it is impermeable to the drug. Thus, bacteria are intrinsically resistant to polyene antibiotics, such as amphotericin B, as sterols that are present in the fungal but not bacterial cell membrane, are the target for these drugs. The lipopolysaccharide outer envelope of Gram-negative bacteria is important in determining susceptibility patterns, since many antibiotics cannot penetrate this barrier to reach their intracellular target. Fortunately, intrinsic resistance is therefore often predictable, and should not pose problems provided that informed and judicious choices of antibiotics are made for the treatment of infection. Of greater concern is the primarily unpredictable acquisition or emergence of resistance in previously susceptible microbes, sometimes during the course of therapy itself.

Acquired resistance

Introduction of clinically effective antibiotics has been followed invariably by the emergence of resistant strains of bacteria among species that would normally be considered to be susceptible. Acquisition of resistance has seriously reduced the therapeutic value of many important antibiotics, but is also a major stimulus to the constant search for new and more effective antimicrobial drugs. However, while the emergence of resistance to new antibiotics is inevitable, the rate of development and spread of resistance is not predictable.

Table 8.1 Effective antimicrobial spectrum of some of the most commonly used antibacterial agents

Organism	Peni-cillins	Cephalo-sporins	Amino-glycosides	Tetra-cyclines	Macro-lides	Chloram-phenicol	Fluoro-quinolones	Sulphon-amides	Trimeth-oprim	Metro-nidazole	Glyco-peptides
Gram-positive bacteria											
Staph. aureus	V	(S)	(S)	(S)	(S)	(S)	V	(S)	(S)	R	S
Str. pyogenes	S	S	R	(S)	S	S	V	(S)	S	R	S
Other streptococci	S	S	R	(S)	S	S	V	(S)	S	R	S
Enterococci	V	R	R	(S)	S	S	V	(S)	(S)	R	(S)
Clostridium spp.	S	S	R	S	S	S	V	(S)	R	S	S
Gram-negative bacteria											
Esch. coli	V	V	(S)	(S)	R	(S)	(S)	(S)	(S)	R	R
Other enterobacteria	V	V	(S)	(S)	R	(S)	(S)	(S)	(S)	R	R
Ps. aeruginosa	V	V	V	R	R	R	(S)	R	R	R	R
H. influenzae	V	V	R	(S)	S	S	S	(S)	(S)	R	R
Neisseria spp.	V	S	R	(S)	S	S	(S)	(S)	R	R	R
Bacteroides spp.	R	V	R	(S)	S	S	V	(S)	R	S	R
Other organisms											
Mycobacteria	R	R	V	R	R	R	(S)	R	R	R	R
Chlamydiae	R	R	R	S	S	S	S	S	S	R	R
Mycoplasmas	R	R	R	S	S	S	S	R	R	R	R
Fungi	R	R	R	R	R	R	R	R	R	R	R

S, usually considered susceptible; R, usually considered resistant; (S), strain variation in susceptibility; V, variation among related drugs and/or strains.

The first systematic observations of acquired drug resistance were made by Paul Ehrlich between 1902 and 1909 while using dyes and organic arsenicals to treat mice infected experimentally with trypanosomes. Within a very few years of the introduction of sulphonamides and penicillin (in 1935 and 1941 respectively), micro-organisms originally susceptible to these drugs were found to have acquired resistance. When penicillin came into use less than 1% of all strains of *Staphylococcus aureus* were resistant to its action. By 1946, however, under the selective pressure of this antibiotic, the proportion of penicillin-resistant strains found in hospitals had risen to 14%. A year later, 38% were resistant, and today, resistance is found in more than 90% of all strains of *Staph. aureus*. In contrast, over the same period, an equally important pathogen, *Streptococcus pyogenes*, has remained uniformly suscep-tible to penicillin, although there is no guarantee that resistance will not spread to *Str. pyogenes* in future years.

There is no clear explanation for the marked differences in rate or extent of acquisition of resistance between different species. Possession of the genetic capacity for resistance does not always explain its prevalence in a particular species. Even when selection pressures are similar, the end result may not be the same. Thus, although about 90% of all strains of *Staph. aureus* are now resistant to penicillin, the same has not happened to ampicillin resistance in *Esch. coli* under similar selection pressure. At present, apart from localized outbreaks involving epidemic strains, about 40–50% of *Esch. coli* strains are resistant to ampicillin, and this level has remained more or less steady for a number of years. However, since an increasing incidence of resistance is at least partly a consequence of selective pressure, it is not surprising that the withdrawal of an antibiotic from clinical use may often result in a slow reduction in the number of resistant strains encountered in a particular environment. For example, fluoroquinolone resistant strains of *Ps. aeruginosa* that emerged in some hospitals as ciprofloxacin or levofloxacin were used more frequently were replaced by more susceptible strains following restriction of removal of these drugs. Conversely, sulphonamide resistant *Esch. coli* strains that became commonplace when the sulphonamide-containing combination drug co-trimoxazole was widely used are still prevalent. This is probably because the selection pressure still exists for other antibiotics, such as ampicillin, and the genes coding for sulphonamide and ampicillin resistance are often closely linked on plasmids; hence, use of one antibiotic can select or maintain resistance to another.

The introduction of new antibiotics has also resulted in changes to the predominant spectrum of organisms responsible for infections. In the 1960s semi-synthetic 'β-lactamase stable' penicillins and cephalosporins were introduced which, temporarily, solved the problem of staphylococcal infections. Unfortunately, Gram-negative bacteria then became the major pathogens found in hospitals and rapidly acquired resistance to multiple antibiotics in the succeeding years. In the 1970s the pendulum swung the other way with the first outbreaks of hospital infection with multiresistant staphylococci that were resistant to nearly all antistaphylococcal agents. Outbreaks of infection caused by such organisms have occurred subsequently all over the world.

There are now signs that Gram-negative bacteria are once again assuming greater importance, particularly in hospitals. Resistance to newer cephalo-sporins—mediated by extended-spectrum β-lactamases—and fluoroquino-lones in *Esch. coli* and other enterobacteria is increasing, rendering these commonly used antibiotics less effective. Multiresistant Gram-negative bacteria (such as *Acinetobacter* species) have emerged that are resistant to most and, occasionally, all approved antibiotics.

Types of acquired resistance

Two main types of acquired resistance may be encountered in bacterial species that would normally be considered susceptible to a particular antibacterial agent.

Mutational resistance

In any large population of bacterial cells a very few individual cells may spontaneously become resistant (see Chapter 10). Such resistant cells have no particular survival advantage in the absence of antibiotic, but after the introduction of antibiotic treatment susceptible bacterial cells will be killed, so that the (initially) very few resistant cells can proliferate until they even-tually form a wholly resistant population. Many antimicrobial agents select for this type of acquired resistance in many different bacterial species, both in vitro and in vivo. The problem has been recognized as being of particular importance in the long-term treatment of tuberculosis with antituberculosis drugs.

Transmissible resistance

A more spectacular type of acquired resistance occurs when genes conferring antibiotic resistance transfer from a resistant bacterial cell to a sensitive one. The simultaneous transfer of resistance to several unrelated antimicrobial agents can be demonstrated readily, both in the laboratory and the patient. Exponential transfer and spread of existing resistance genes through a previ-ously susceptible bacterial population is a much more efficient mechanism of acquiring resistance than the development of resistance by mutation of individual susceptible cells.

Mechanisms by which transfer of resistance genes takes place are discussed in Chapter 10. Here it is sufficient to stress that however resistance appears in a hitherto susceptible bacterial cell or population, resistance will only become widespread under the selective pressures produced by the presence of appropriate antibiotics. Also, the development of resistant cells does not have to happen often or on a large scale. A single mutation or transfer event can, if the appropriate selective pressures are operating, lead to the replacement of a susceptible population by a resistant one. Without selective pressure, antibiotic resistance may be a handicap rather than an asset to a bacterium.

Cross-resistance and multiple resistance

These terms are often confused. Cross-resistance involves resistance to a number of different members of a group of (usually) chemically related agents that are affected alike by the same resistance mechanism. For example, there is almost complete cross-resistance between the different tetracyclines, because tetracycline resistance results largely from an efflux mechanism that affects all members of the group. The situation is more complex among other antibiotic families. Thus, resistance to aminoglycosides may be mediated by any one of a number of different drug-inactivating enzymes (see Table 9.3, p. 135) with different substrate specificities, and the range of aminoglycosides to which the organism is resistant will depend on which enzyme it produces. Cross-resistance can also be observed occasionally between unrelated antibiotics. For example, a change in the outer membrane structure of Gram-negative bacilli may concomitantly deny access of unrelated compounds to their target sites.

In contrast, multiple drug (multidrug) resistance involves a bacterium becoming resistant to several unrelated antibiotics by different resistance mechanisms. For example, if a staphylococcus is resistant to penicillin, gentamicin, and tetracycline, the resistances must have originated independently, since the strain destroys the penicillin with a β-lactamase, inactivates gentamicin with an aminoglycoside-modifying enzyme, and excludes tetracycline from the cell by an active efflux mechanism.

It is, however, not always clear whether cross-resistance or multiple resistance is being observed. Genes conferring resistance to several unrelated agents can be transferred en bloc from one bacterial cell to another on plasmids (see Chapter 10), thereby giving the appearance of cross-resistance.

In such cases, detailed biochemical and genetic analysis may be required to prove that the resistance mechanisms are distinct (multiple resistance), although the genes conferring resistance are linked and transferred together on one plasmid.

The clinical problem of drug resistance

Concerns about resistance have been raised at regular intervals since the first introduction of antimicrobial chemotherapy, but awareness of the antibiotic resistance problem has probably never been greater than it is today. It has been suggested that antibiotic resistance is becoming so commonplace that there is a danger of returning to the pre-antibiotic era. It is important not to understate or overstate the problem; the situation is presently becoming serious, but is not yet desperate since most infections are still treatable with several currently available agents. This may, however, mean that the only antibiotics that are still active are more toxic or less effective (or both) than those to which bacteria have acquired resistance. For example, it is generally accepted that glycopeptide antibiotics are less effective in the treatment of *Staph. aureus* infection than are antistaphylococcal penicillins (e.g. flucloxacillin); since the latter cannot be used against methicillin-resistant *Staph. aureus* (MRSA), this may partly explain the poorer outcome that is seen in such cases in comparison with infection caused by methicillin-susceptible strains.

There is good evidence that if the antibiotic regimen chosen is subsequently shown to be inactive against the pathogens causing infection, then patient outcome is worse (Fig. 8.1). This means that clinicians are likely to opt for unnecessarily broad-spectrum therapy particularly in critically ill patients. Unfortunately, repeated use of such regimens against bacteria that harbour resistance genes intensifies the selective pressure for further resistance development, notably in hospital, where the most vulnerable patients are managed.

In many less-developed countries of the world the therapeutic options may be severely restricted for economic reasons. There is no doubt that the problem of antibiotic resistance is a global issue, and in future years there is a real possibility that physicians will be faced increasingly with infections for which effective treatment is not available. Some of the organisms in which resistance is a particular problem are summarized below.

Enteric Gram-negative bacteria

The prevalence of resistance in hospital strains of enteric Gram-negative bacteria has been rising steadily for the past 40 years, particularly in

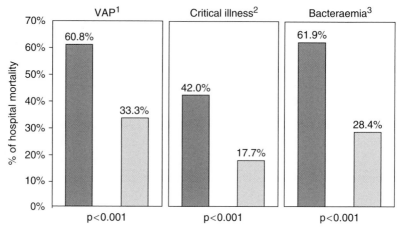

Fig. 8.1 Mortality recorded in three separate studies for patients who received antibiotic treatment that was subsequently shown to be inactive (dark grey) or active (light grey) against pathogens isolated. VAP, ventilator associated pneumonia. Data from: [1]Kollef MH, Ward S. The influence of mini-BAL cultures on patient outcomes: implications for the antibiotic management of ventilator-associated pneumonia. *Chest* 1998; **113**: 412–420; [2]Kollef MH Sherman G, Ward S, Fraser VJ Inadequate antimicrobial treatment of infections: a risk factor for hospital mortality among critically ill patients. *Chest* 1999; **115**: 462–474; [3]Ibrahim EH, Sherman G, Ward S, Fraser VJ, Kollef MH. The influence of inadequate antimicrobial treatment of bloodstream infections on patient outcomes in the ICU setting. *Chest* 2000; **118**: 146–155.

large units. Although cephalosporins, quinolones, and aminoglycosides have been developed to cope with the problem, resistance to these newer compounds continues to increase in most countries. Outbreaks of infection caused by multiresistant *Klebsiella* strains and extended-spectrum β-lactamase-producing enterobacteria in general are being reported with worrying frequency, especially in high dependency areas of hospitals.

Widespread resistance in enteric bacteria is a particular problem in less-developed areas of the world where heavy and indiscriminate use of antibiotics may combine with a high prevalence of drug-resistant bacteria in the faecal flora, poor standards of sanitation, and a high incidence of diarrhoeal disease to encourage the rapid emergence and spread of multiresistant strains of enteric bacteria. Epidemics of diarrhoeal disease caused by multiresistant strains of intestinal pathogens, including *Vibrio cholerae*, shigellae, salmonellae, and toxin-producing strains of *Esch. coli*, have occurred around the world.

modification performed, and by the site of modification on the aminoglycoside molecule. Over 30 such modifying enzymes and their variants have been identified by biochemical or nucleic acid-based methods, and these can be divided into three main groups: aminoglycoside acetylating enzymes; nucleotidyltransferase enzymes; and phosphorylating enzymes. Examples of the most widely distributed enzymes are listed in Table 9.3.

Figure 9.3 shows the structure of kanamycin A, a typical aminoglycoside, and indicates the various sites at which modification can take place. The presence or absence of available amino or hydroxyl groupings affects the susceptibility to various enzymes; this is the basis of variability within the aminoglycoside group. The steric configuration of the groupings is also important; thus, the semisynthetic aminoglycoside amikacin is, structurally,

Table 9.3 Examples of some of the most common aminoglycoside-modifying enzymes and their characteristic substrates

Enzyme	Typical substrates	Bacterial distribution	
		Gram-positive	Gram-negative
Acetyltransferases			
AAC (3)-I	Gen	−	+
AAC (3)-II	Gen, Tob, Net	−	+
AAC (3)-IV	Gen, Tob, Net	−	+
AAC (2′)	Gen, Tob	−	+
AAC (6′)-I	Tob, Amk, Net, Kan	+	+
AAC (6′)-II	Gen, Tob, Net	−	+
Nucleotidyltransferases			
ANT (4′)	Tob, Amk, Kan, Neo	+	(−)
ANT (2″)	Gen, Tob, Kan	−	+
Phosphotransferases			
APH (3′)-III	Kan, Neo	+	−
APH (3′)-VI	Neo, Kan, Amk	+	+
APH (2″)	Gen, Tob, Kan	+	−

(−) indicates that this activity is uncommon. Amk, amikacin; Gen, gentamicin; Kan, kanamycin; Neo, neomycin; Net, netilmicin; Tob, tobramycin. The figure in brackets indicates the site of modification according to the internationally accepted numbering system for the various parts of the complex aminoglycoside molecule (see Fig. 9.2).

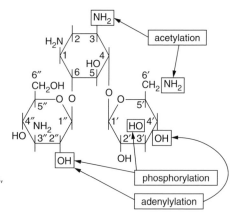

Fig. 9.3 Structure of kanamycin A, showing the sites at which enzymic modification can occur.

related closely to kanamycin A, but is much less susceptible to enzymic modification because of a hydroxyaminobutyric acid side chain that alters the steric configuration of the molecule. The acetylating enzymes, of which there are at least 16 types, catalyse the transfer of acetate from acetyl coenzyme A to an amino group on the aminoglycoside molecule. These enzymes modify only deoxystreptamine-containing aminoglycosides (p. 36) and are, therefore, without effect on streptomycin or spectinomycin. By contrast, aminoglycoside nucleotidyltransferases use adenosine triphosphate or other nucleotides as substrates and attach the nucleotide to exposed hydroxyl groups, while phosphotransferases also modify hydroxyl groups, but by attachment of a phosphate molecule.

Various patterns of cross-resistance can be shown by bacteria that produce different enzymes (Table 9.3), but these are complicated further because many clinical isolates produce more than one enzyme at any one time. Susceptibility or resistance to any one agent cannot be predicted reliably from results obtained for another; thus, susceptibility tests must be performed with the agent that is to be used therapeutically.

Although aminoglycosides exhibit poor activity against enterococci, they interact synergically with β-lactam antibiotics to achieve a more rapid and complete bactericidal action. Unfortunately plasmid-mediated high-level aminoglycoside resistance, which abolishes synergy, has become much more prevalent in enterococci, so removing the possibility of synergistic β-lactam–aminoglycoside therapy in serious enterococcal infection caused by such strains.

When the aminoglycoside-modifying enzymes were first described, they were considered to be examples of drug-inactivating enzymes analogous to those responsible for resistance to β-lactam antibiotics and chloramphenicol. However, aminoglycoside-modifying enzymes mediate resistance by modifying only small amounts of antibiotic. They are strategically placed near the inner cytoplasmic membrane where they are accessible to acetyl coenzyme A and adenosine triphosphate. As soon as a few molecules of drug are modified, all further transport of drug into the cell becomes blocked.

Chloramphenicol

Resistance to chloramphenicol in both Gram-positive and Gram-negative bacteria is normally associated with production of an enzyme, chloramphenicol acetyltransferase, which converts the drug to either the monoacetate or diacetate. The acetylated drug will not bind to the bacterial ribosome, and so cannot block protein synthesis. Several different acetyltransferases have been described. Some appear to be genus- and species-specific; others, usually plasmid or transposon-associated, are more widespread. This variety is a little surprising since chloramphenicol has been used less widely than many other antibiotics because of its rare, but serious, toxic side effects.

Alteration or protection of the target site

Resistance arising from the selection of rare, pre-existent mutants from within an otherwise susceptible bacterial population has been described for many antibiotics. The mutations usually affect the drug target and often confer high-level resistance in a single step. The emergence of this type of resistance during therapy is an important cause of treatment failure with certain drugs, including rifampicin, the older quinolones, fusidic acid, and various antituberculosis drugs. Use of combinations of antibiotics can prevent the emergence of such resistance during therapy, since the likelihood of independent mutations conferring resistance to two or more unrelated antibiotics appearing simultaneously in the same cell is very small. This strategy has been crucial in antituberculosis therapy. Similarly, monotherapy of staphylococcal infection with rifampicin or fusidic acid should not normally be used.

Variants exhibiting low levels of resistance to almost any antibiotic can be isolated readily from most bacteria. In contrast to single-step mutants they usually develop in a stepwise fashion, and may be accompanied by other phenotypic changes (e.g. slower growth rate, colonial variation on solid media, reduced virulence). These so-called 'fitness costs' become more marked as the degree of resistance increases. It is likely that the shifts in penicillin susceptibility of gonococci and pneumococci that have occurred over the years result from such cumulative changes.

β-Lactam antibiotics

The major mechanism of resistance to β-lactam antibiotics is enzymic inactivation (see above), but mechanisms involving target site modification also occur. *Streptococcus pneumoniae* strains with reduced susceptibility to penicillin exhibit alterations in the target penicillin-binding proteins (PBPs; p. 29) that result in reduced ability to bind penicillin. Similarly, methicillin resistance in staphylococci is associated with the synthesis of a modified PBP (PBP 2′), which exhibits decreased affinity for methicillin and other β-lactam antibiotics. Low-level resistance to penicillin in *N. gonorrhoeae* has also been associated with alterations to PBPs. Such resistance appears to have developed by rare mutational events and to have become disseminated as a result of considerable antibiotic selection pressure.

Glycopeptides

Resistance to vancomycin and teicoplanin first emerged in enterococci only after the antibiotic had been available for 30 years. Expression of resistance depends on the presence or absence of several genes and two enzymes (a ligase and a dehydrogenase), which probably originated in non-human pathogens and were transferred to enterococci. The net effect of these is target site alteration. Glycopeptides bind to the D-alanyl-D-alanine terminus of the muramyl pentapeptide of peptidoglycan (p. 31). Enterococci that exhibit high-level resistance to glycopeptides produce a new dipeptide terminus, either D-alanyl-D-lactate or D-alanyl-D-serine. Such substitutions allow cell wall synthesis to continue in the presence of one or both of the currently available glycopeptides, vancomycin and teicoplanin. Several different glycopeptide resistance phenotypes have been described (Table 9.4). Glycopeptide resistance is usually inducible in those strains that posses the necessary genes and enzymes, but some essentially non-pathogenic enterococci (e.g. *Enterococcus gallinarum*, *E. casseliflavus*, and *E. flavescens*) are constitutively resistant to low-moderate levels of vancomycin.

The mechanism of the low-level resistance to glycopeptide antibiotics that has emerged in some *Staph. aureus* and coagulase-negative staphylococci has not been completely elucidated, but appears to be associated with overproduction of peptidoglycan precursors that require increased amounts of drug to saturate them. Very rare strains of *Staph. aureus* that are highly

caused by loss of porins, sometimes exacerbated by β-lactamase production; e.g. imipenem resistance in *Ps. aeruginosa*.

Chloramphenicol

A few strains of chloramphenicol-resistant Gram-negative bacilli possess a plasmid that appears to confer the property of impermeability to chloramphenicol upon the host cell.

Quinolones

Gram-negative bacteria have been described in which resistance to quinolones is caused by impermeability associated with a decrease in the amount of the OmpF outer membrane porin protein. Such strains may simultaneously acquire resistance to β-lactam antibiotics and some other agents that gain access through the OmpF porin. Resistance caused by active efflux also occurs in some Gram-negative bacilli and staphylococci. This can be mediated by efflux pumps that are specific for quinolones or by non-specific transporter pumps.

Aminoglycosides

A mechanism of resistance to aminoglycosides, unrelated to enzymic modification, is associated with alterations in membrane proteins that affect active transport of the antibiotic into the cell.

Metabolic bypass

Most common resistance mechanisms can be accommodated in one or other of the three major groups described already. However, there are two known examples in which a plasmid or transposon provides the cell with an entirely new and drug-resistant enzyme that can bypass the susceptible chromosomal enzyme that is also present unaltered in the cell.

Sulphonamides

Sulphonamides exert their bacteristatic effect by competitive inhibition of dihydropteroate synthetase. Sulphonamide-resistant strains of Gram-negative bacilli synthesize an additional dihydropteroate synthetase that is unaffected by sulphonamides. The additional enzyme allows continued functioning of the threatened metabolic pathway in the presence of the drug. At least two such enzymes are widespread in Gram-negative bacilli throughout the world.

Trimethoprim

Trimethoprim blocks a later step in the same metabolic pathway by inhibiting the dihydrofolate reductase enzymes in susceptible bacteria. Resistant strains synthesize a new, trimethoprim-insensitive, dihydrofolate reductase as well as the normal drug-susceptible chromosomal enzyme. At least 14 groups of trimethoprim-insusceptible dihydrofolate reductases have been described in Gram-negative bacilli, and a further example is found in multiresistant isolates of *Staph. aureus.*

The mechanisms discussed above illustrate the diversity of ways in which microbes can become resistant to the drugs deployed against them. However, any attempt to limit the spread of drug resistance requires not only knowledge of the mechanisms themselves, but also an understanding of the genetic factors that control their emergence and continued evolution. These factors are the subject of the next chapter.

Chapter 10

Genetics of resistance

All the properties of a microbial cell, including those of medical importance such as antibiotic resistance and virulence determinants, are determined ultimately by the microbial genome, which in turn comprises the three sources of genetic information in the cell: the chromosome, plasmids, and bacteriophages. Resistance of bacteria to antibiotics may be either intrinsic or acquired (see Chapter 8). Intrinsic resistance is the 'natural' resistance possessed by a bacterial species and is usually specified by chromosomal genes. An example of a bacterial species with a high degree of intrinsic resistance is *Pseudomonas aeruginosa*. By contrast, acquired resistance occurs in formerly susceptible cells, either following alterations to the existing genome or by transfer of genetic information between cells. Thus, a basic knowledge of microbial genetics is essential to understand the development and spread of resistance to antimicrobial drugs.

The heritable information that specifies a bacterial cell, and passes to daughter cells at cell division, is carried in bacteria, as in all living cells, as an ordered sequence of nucleotide pairs along molecules of DNA. The process of transcription of this information into messenger RNA, and its subsequent translation into functioning proteins by ribosomes, is also similar in bacteria and in other cells.

The bacterial chromosome

The main source of genetic information in a bacterial cell is the chromosome. Each bacterial cell has a single chromosome, which, in the vast majority of cases, is known to form a single closed circular DNA molecule. In *Escherichia coli*, the organism studied most intensively, this single DNA molecule comprises about 4×10^3 kb (kilobases) and is about 1.4 mm in length. Considering the average cell is about 1–3 µm in length, only by 'super-coiling' of DNA can the chromosome fit inside the bacterium. Enzymes known as DNA gyrases control the process of super-coiling DNA. Conversely, DNA uncoiling, which is necessary for messenger RNA production or chromosome replication, is controlled by DNA topoisomerases.

The chromosome is found in the cytoplasm of the cell, not separated from it by a nuclear membrane. Transcription of DNA and translation of the resulting messenger RNA can therefore proceed simultaneously. Most bacterial chromosomes contain sufficient DNA to encode for 1000–3000 different genes. Not all of these genes need to be expressed at any one time, and indeed it would be wasteful for the cell to do so. Gene regulation is therefore necessary, and this can occur at either the transcriptional or translational level.

Chromosomal mutations to antibiotic resistance

Mutations result from rare mistakes in the DNA replication process and occur at the rate of between 10^{-4} and 10^{-10} per cell division. They usually involve deletion, substitution, or addition of one or only a few base pairs, which cause an alteration in the amino acid composition of a specific protein. Such mistakes are random and spontaneous. They occur continuously in cell genes and are independent of the presence or absence of a particular antibiotic. The vast majority of mutations are repaired by the cell without any noticeable effect. In the presence of an antibiotic some of these occasional spontaneous antibiotic-resistant mutants that are present in a large susceptible population of bacteria may be selected. In such a situation, the susceptible cells will be killed or inhibited by the antibiotic, whereas the resistant mutants will survive and proliferate to become the predominant type. Most chromosomal resistance mutations result in alterations to permeability or specific antibiotic target sites, but some result in enhanced production of an inactivating enzyme or bypass mechanism. The latter types are mutations at the transcriptional or translational level in gene regulatory mechanisms.

Chromosomal mutations to antibiotic resistance can be divided into single-step and multi-step types.

Single large-step mutations

With these mutations, a single mutational change results in a large increase in the minimum inhibitory concentration of a particular antibiotic. Single-step mutations may lead to treatment failure when these drugs are used alone. In some Gram-negative bacilli, mutations in the genetic regulatory system for the normally low-level chromosomal β-lactamase may result in a vast overproduction (sometimes referred to as 'derepression') of this enzyme with resulting slow hydrolysis of compounds such as cefotaxime and ceftazidime that are considered under normal circumstances to be β-lactamase stable.

Multistep (stepwise) mutations

These are sequential mutations that result in cumulative gradual stepwise increases in the minimum inhibitory concentration of a particular antibiotic. They are clinically quite common, especially in situations where only low concentrations of antibiotic can be delivered to the site of an infection.

Plasmids

The bacterial chromosome carries all the genes necessary for the survival and replication of the bacterial cell under most circumstances. Many, perhaps all, bacteria also carry additional molecules of DNA (usually between 2 and 200 kb in size) known as plasmids, which are separate from, and normally replicate independently of, the bacterial chromosome. Plasmids can carry genes that confer a wide range of properties on the cells that carry them. In general, these are properties that are not essential for the survival of the cell under normal circumstances, but which offer the cells a survival advantage in unusual or adverse conditions. Examples of such properties are:

* fertility: the ability to conjugate with and transfer genetic information into other bacteria (see later)
* resistance to antibiotics: antibiotic resistance encountered clinically is often associated with plasmids
* ability to produce bacteriocins: proteins inhibitory to other bacteria that may be ecological competitors
* exotoxin production
* immunity to some bacteriophages
* ability to use unusual sugars and other substrates as foods.

Plasmids differ in size, DNA base composition, the DNA fragments that can be recognized after treatment with restriction endonucleases ('plasmid fingerprints'), and in their incompatibility behaviour. Compatible plasmids can coexist in the same host cell, while incompatible plasmids cannot, and so tend to be unstable and displace one another. There are at least 20 incompatibility (Inc) groups within the plasmids found in enteric Gram-negative bacilli, and similar incompatibility schemes are used to subdivide staphylococcal plasmids and those found in *Pseudomonas* spp.

Bacteriophages

The third possible source of genetic information in a bacterial cell is a bacteriophage. Bacteriophages (phages) are viruses that infect bacteria.

Most phages will attack only a relatively small number of strains of related bacteria—they have a narrow and specific host range. Phages can be divided into two main types:

• Virulent phages inevitably destroy by lysis any bacteria that they infect, with the release of numerous new phage particles from each lysed cell.

• Temperate (lysogenic) phages may either lyse or lysogenize infected bacterial cells. In the state of lysogeny, the phage nucleic acid is replicated in a stable and dormant fashion within the infected cell, often following insertion into the host cell chromosome. Such a dormant phage is known as a prophage. However, while in the prophage state, some prophage genes may be expressed and may confer additional properties on the cell. Once in every few thousand cell divisions, a prophage becomes released from the dormant state and enters the lytic cycle, with subsequent destruction of its host cell and release of new phage particles into the surrounding medium.

The possibility of using naturally occurring phages for the treatment of some infections (phage therapy) has been suggested, partly in response to the threat posed by antibiotic resistance pathogens.

Transfer of genetic information

There are three ways in which genetic information can be transferred from one bacterial cell into another: transformation, transduction, and conjugation.

• Transformation involves lysis of a bacterial cell and the release of naked DNA into the surrounding medium. Under certain circumstances, intact bacterial cells in the vicinity can acquire some of this DNA. This process has been much studied in the laboratory, but there are few convincing demonstrations of its occurrence in vivo. The process depends crucially on the ability of the recipient cells to be competent for uptake of free DNA.

• Transduction involves the accidental incorporation of bacterial DNA, either from the chromosome or a plasmid, into a bacteriophage particle during the phage lytic cycle. The phage particle then acts as a vector and transfers the bacterial DNA to the next cell that it infects.

• Conjugation involves physical contact between two bacterial cells. The cells adhere to one another and DNA passes unidirectionally from one cell, termed the donor, into the other, the recipient. Ability to conjugate depends on carriage of an appropriate plasmid or transposon (see later) by the host cell.

These transfer mechanisms means that bacteria do not have to rely solely on a process of mutation and selection for their evolution. They can, therefore, acquire and express blocks of genetic information that have evolved elsewhere. A bacterial cell can, for example, acquire by conjugation a plasmid that carries genes conferring resistance to several different antibiotics. As a result, within a very short time following the receipt of such a plasmid by a susceptible cell, the bacteria in a given niche may change from being predominantly susceptible to being resistant to multiple drugs. Of course, the ability to transfer genes in this way does not eliminate the need for these to evolve; however, once they have evolved, it ensures their eventual widespread dissemination under appropriate selection pressures.

Evolution of new resistance gene combinations

The distinction between chromosomal and plasmid genes is not absolute. Where appropriate regions of DNA homology exist, classic ('normal' or 'homologous') recombination can occur, both between different plasmids and between plasmids and the chromosome. Although this process can lead to the formation of new antibiotic resistance gene combinations, it is relatively uncommon in bacteria because there are few regions of sequence homology between the bacterial chromosome and plasmids that can be exploited for this purpose. Homologous recombination is used by researchers to create 'knockout' cells in which the function of a specific gene is disrupted. A more important mechanism by which antibiotic resistance genes can pass naturally from one bacterial replicon to another is the 'illegitimate' recombination process known as transposition.

Transposons

Transposition depends on the existence of specific genetic elements termed transposons. These elements are discrete sequences of DNA capable of translocation (transposition) from one replicon (plasmid or chromosome) to another. Unlike classic ('normal') recombination, transposons do not share extensive regions of homology with the replicon into which they insert. In many cases, transposons consist of individual resistance genes, or groups of genes, bounded by DNA sequences called either direct or inverted repeats, i.e. a sequence of bases at one end of the transposon that also appears, either in direct or reverse order, at the other end. These repeats may be relatively short, often of the order of 40 base pairs, but longer examples have been identified. It is likely that these DNA sequences provide highly specific recognition sites for certain enzymes (transposases) that catalyse the movement of transposons from one replicon to another, without the need for extensive regions of sequence homology. Depending upon the transposon involved, insertion may occur at only a few or at many different sites on the host replicon. Transposons may carry genes conferring resistance to many different antibiotics, as well as other metabolic properties, and their existence helps to explain how a single antibiotic resistance gene can become disseminated over a wide range of unrelated replicons.

Isolated DNA sequences analogous to the terminal sequences of transposons can also move from one replicon to another, or be inserted in any region of any DNA molecule. Such insertion sequences appear to contain only genes that are related to insertion functions; however, in principle at least, two similar insertion sequences could bracket any assemblage of genes and convert it into a transposon. Thus, theoretically, all replicons are accessible to transposition and all genes are potentially transposable. This theory is of crucial evolutionary importance since it explains how genes of appropriate function can accumulate on a single replicon under the impact of selection pressure. Transposons and insertion sequences therefore play a vital part in plasmid evolution.

Integrons

Transposons may contain combinations of genes conferring resistance to various different antibiotics. An important question concerns the mechanism by which new combinations of antibiotic resistance genes are formed. It is now apparent that special molecular structures, termed integrons, may enable the formation of new combinations of resistance genes within a bacterial cell, either on a plasmid or within a transposon, in response to selection pressures.

Integrons appear to consist of two conserved segments of DNA located either side of inserted antibiotic resistance genes. Individual resistance genes seem to be capable of insertion or removal as 'cassettes' between these conserved structures. The cassettes can be found inserted in different orders and combinations. Integrons also act as an expression vector for 'foreign' antibiotic resistance genes by supplying a promoter for transcription of cassettes derived originally from completely unrelated organisms. Integrons lack many of the features associated with transposons, including direct or inverted repeats and functions required for transposition. They do, however, possess site-specific integration functions, notably a special enzyme termed an integrase.

The precise role of integrons in the evolution and spread of antibiotic resistance genes remains to be determined, but they have been found, together with their associated antibiotic resistance gene cassettes, in many different Gram-negative bacteria. At least three potential mechanisms of spread exist:

- the potential mobility of an integron itself by site-specific insertion;
- spread following insertion of an integron into a transposon;
- horizontal transfer of integrons on plasmids.

Whatever the mechanism, unrelated clinical isolates from different worldwide locations have been shown to carry the same integron structures, and it seems that these structures may play a key role in the formation and dissemination of new combinations of antibiotic resistance genes.

The process of evolution and spread of antibiotic resistance genes continues. The origin of resistance genes carried by integrons, transposons, or plasmids, or even the origin of these elements themselves, is generally not known, but it has been possible to observe a steady increase in the numbers of resistant bacterial strains following the introduction of successive chemotherapeutic agents into clinical use. There are many examples and the evolutionary process is a continuous event. The *qnrA* genes that encode plasmid mediated quinolone resistance are embedded in complex integrons. Similar genes have been identified in the water-borne species *Shewanella algae*, so emphasizing the potential for spread of resistance mechanisms from environmental bacteria.

Genotypic resistance

To summarize the earlier discussion, genes conferring resistance to antibiotics are often found inserted into integrons, and may be part of the bacterial chromosome or may be carried on plasmids, transposons, or as part of a phage genome. The distribution of these genes between the chromosome and other elements reflects to some extent the biochemical mechanisms involved. For example, resistance that results from mutational alteration of an existing target protein will normally be chromosomal in location and will not be integron-associated, whereas resistance genes for entirely new enzymes, such as the aminoglycoside-modifying enzymes, novel β-lactamases, or trimethoprim-resistant dihydrofolate reductases, are commonly carried on plasmids and transposons as part of integrons. This reflects the fact that the evolution of any new enzyme is likely to be a very long process; the occurrence of the genes for such enzymes on plasmids, transposons, and integrons enables spread of these genes between different strains, species, and genera rather than requiring evolution of the genes afresh by each bacterial strain for itself. The discovery of a variant gene encoding an aminoglycoside modifying (acetyltransferase) enzyme that can mediate quinolone resistance has highlighted the plasticity of resistance mechanisms. In this case, the new mechanism is all the more startling given that antimicrobial-modifying enzymes have traditionally been antibiotic class specific.

Chromosomal and plasmid-mediated types of resistance may be equally important in the antibiotic management of an individual patient. However, the plasmid-encoded variety has achieved greater notoriety because of the spectacular fashion in which bacteria may acquire resistance to a number of unrelated agents by a single genetic event. Furthermore, the potential for spread of plasmid borne resistance to other species or genera highlights the importance of control of pathogens that are antibiotic resistant by virtue of such plasmid genes. Certainly, it has been plasmid-encoded resistance that has caused most problems in the highly selective environment of the hospital. Nevertheless, mutational resistance involving the bacterial chromosome is also a common cause of treatment failure with some compounds. Antibacterial agents for which resistance is not known to be encoded on plasmids (e.g. rifampicin) generally suffer from mutational resistance problems instead.

Phenotypic resistance

So far as is known, phenotypic resistance to antibacterial agents is rare, although it is not always possible to be sure that phenotypic changes brought about in the microenvironment of a lesion do not contribute to insusceptibility of bacteria in the infected host. In the laboratory, phenotypic resistance can sometimes be induced; for example, varying the conditions of growth of *Ps. aeruginosa* can alter the outer envelope, and this affects susceptibility to polymyxins.

Another example is the failure of penicillins and cephalosporins to kill 'persisters' (those cells in a bacterial population that survive exposure to concentrations of β-lactam agents lethal to the rest of the culture). This does not result from a genetic event since the resistance is not heritable, and it is probable that the 'resistant' bacteria are caught in a particular metabolic state at the time of first encounter with the drug.

A peculiar form of phenotypic resistance is observed with mecillinam, a β-lactam antibiotic which, unusually, does not affect bacterial cell division.

Mecillinam induces surface changes in susceptible Gram-negative bacilli which generally lead to cell death by osmotic rupture (p. 29). However, those cells in the population that happen to have low internal osmolality survive, and, as mecillinam lacks the ability to prevent growth and division, such bacteria continue to grow in a morphologically altered form. On withdrawal of the drug, the bacteria resume their normal shape and, in due course, revert to the same mixed susceptibility as the original parent culture.

The influence of antibiotic selection pressure

Antibiotic resistance genes, and the genetic elements that carry them, existed before the introduction of antibiotics into human medicine. However, it is clear that the emergence and survival of predominantly resistant bacterial populations is due to the selective pressure associated with the widespread use of antibiotics. Resistant cells survive in a given niche at the expense of susceptible cells of the same or other species. In some cases, however, there is a fitness cost to resistant bacterial cells that may mean that they are less able to compete once the selective pressure imparted by the antibiotic is removed. In such cases, any antibiotic susceptible progeny cells that remain may be counterselected in preference to these unfit mutants. Individual cells may lose their plasmids and chromosomal mutations may revert to being antibiotic susceptible. The implications of this process for efforts to control and limit the spread of bacterial drug resistance are discussed in the next chapter.

Chapter 11

Control of the spread of resistance

The 60-year period during which antibiotics have been available has seen dramatic changes in the disease burden caused by infections. Outcomes from infections such as pneumococcal pneumonia, tuberculosis, and streptococcal puerperal sepsis, that used to cause considerable morbidity and mortality, are now frequently benign, at least in developed countries. We can also prevent much infection by using antibiotics during high-risk procedures, notably in the peri-operative period. The immense social, economic, and health benefits that are due to antibiotic use are, however, increasingly overshadowed by the issue of resistance. Indeed, the emergence and spread of multiresistant strains (sometimes referred to emotively as 'superbugs') have raised the spectre of untreatable infection. The reality is that such instances remain extremely rare. However, resistance does limit antibiotic choice available to prescribers, sometimes meaning that less effective, more toxic or more expensive drugs have to be used. For example, the antibiotics needed to treat multiresistant forms of tuberculosis are over 100 times more expensive than the first-line drugs used to treat disease caused by fully susceptible strains. Such excess costs mean that some infections can no longer be treated in poor communities where resistance to first-line drugs is widespread. Furthermore, significant slowing in the development of genuinely new antibiotics (i.e. those with novel modes of action to which cross-resistance to older agents does not occur) has increased the potential for this threat to become a reality that once again compromises patient outcome.

In 1945 during his Nobel Prize acceptance speech Sir Alexander Fleming said 'It is not difficult to make microbes resistant to penicillin in the laboratory by exposing them to concentrations not sufficient to kill them, and the same thing has occasionally happened in the body.' This warning was evident less than a decade after the introduction of penicillin, when a particular penicillin-resistant *Staphylococcus aureus* strain started to cause outbreaks of postoperative and perinatal infection in hospitals across the world. Poor hospital cleaning, increasing dependence on antibiotics and changing healthcare practices were blamed. Unfortunately, these issues are again topical, with frequent media headlines about 'superbugs' and their spread.

Compared with most other drugs of similar potency, antibiotics are remarkably safe, and they are also remarkably effective. This has inevitably led to liberal, even lavish use, and concern has frequently been expressed that excessive and inappropriate use of these agents is the chief cause of the widespread emergence of resistant organisms. Misuse of most drugs tends to have consequences only for the individual patient. Unfortunately, inappropriate antibiotic use can have adverse consequences for both the individual and for wider populations. Figure 11.1 shows the disturbing relationship between the prescribing of penicillin-like antibiotics in multiple populations and the respective prevalence of pneumococcal strains with reduced susceptibility (or frank resistance) to penicillin. Of course, many of the antibiotics prescribed would not have been specifically for pneumococcal infection. This is, therefore, evidence of the selective pressure for resistance emergence in (respiratory tract) flora and subsequent spread of bacteria within populations. Such effects have been referred to as the collateral damage associated with antibiotic therapy.

Availability of antibiotics

Most developed countries have tightly regulated systems for the control of the manufacture, importation, distribution, sale, supply and description of medicinal products, including antibiotics, for human and veterinary use (see Chapter 32). In the global market for medicines, licensing authorities will increasingly be required to ensure that there is a consistency of approach to medicines availability. Currently there are many examples of inconsistencies in the availability and recommendations for use of antibiotics throughout both the developed and developing world. The availability of antibiotics, notably newer more expensive agents is an issue in poorer countries. Pharmaceutical companies have a part to play in helping to ensure that antimicrobial agents, including critical antimalarial, antituberculosis, and antiretroviral drugs are priced and advertised appropriately in these markets.

While the sale and distribution of antibiotics are fairly tightly controlled in rich, developed countries, the marketing of these agents is much less restricted in the poorer, and numerically much larger, developing world. Paradoxically, the use of antibiotics in the developing countries needs to be extended, not restricted, if standards of health are to be brought up to those of the developed world. A key issue here is unregulated 'over the counter' availability of antibiotics. Controversy persists about striking a balance between making effective medicines available in a timely fashion to those who need them, against the potential detrimental effects of uncontrolled

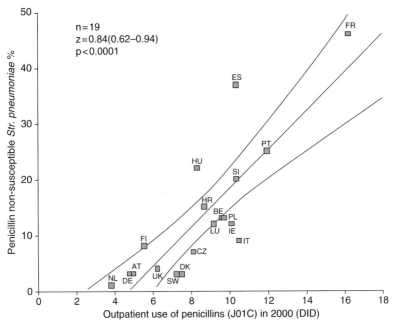

Fig. 11.1 Correlation between antimicrobial use (outpatient prescribing of penicillins) and resistance (prevalence of penicillin-non-susceptible *Str. pneumoniae*) in 19 countries in Europe. Reprinted from: Goossens H, Ferech M, Vander Stichele R, Elseviers M. Outpatient antibiotic use in Europe and association with resistance: a cross-national database study. *Lancet* 2005; **365**: 579–587 with permission from Elsevier.

AT	Austria	NL	Netherlands	DE	Germany
HR	Croatia	SI	Slovenia	IE	Ireland
DK	Denmark	UK	England only	LU	Luxembourg
FR	France	BE	Belgium	PL	Poland
HU	Hungary	CZ	Czech Republic	ES	Spain
IT	Italy	FI	Finland	SW	Sweden
PT	Portugal				

J01C, Systemic antibacterial agents use based on either distribution or reimbursement data; DID: The defined daily dose per 1000 inhabitants daily.

or indiscriminate use. This argument is most pertinent in the case of antimicrobial drugs, as there is no other example in therapeutics in which local misuse of an efficacious agent can lead to a general diminution in its effectiveness. It was no great surprise that chloramphenicol-resistant typhoid bacilli first emerged in South America and penicillin-resistant gonococci in south-east Asia, where unrestricted availability of antibiotics is common-place. In some countries antibiotics can still be purchased easily as single tablets resulting in inappropriate use, suboptimal dosing and the consequent encouragement of resistance.

In the UK fluconazole and aciclovir have been available for over-the-counter purchase without the need for a prescription for more than a decade. There is no convincing evidence that this availability additional to prescribed courses has increased the emergence of resistance to these agents in the target pathogens—*Candida albicans* and herpes simplex virus—for which they are commonly used. This may, however, reflect inherent properties of these drugs uncommonly to select for resistant variants. There is pressure to extend the availability of over-the-counter antibiotics to include drugs such as trimeth-oprim for use in urinary tract infections. It will be important to monitor any such changes closely to determine the benefits and drawbacks of any such deregulation of antibiotics. A related issue is the extension of capacity to prescribe antibiotics (and other drugs) to other healthcare professionals, including pharmacists and nurses. Such extended roles clearly need to be underpinned by appropriate training and education, and the availability of carefully constructed guidelines (see below).

Inappropriate antibiotic use

Attention has repeatedly been drawn to the worldwide public health problem of the spread and persistence of drug-resistant organisms, and there have been frequent calls for regulation to curb the unnecessary use and misuse of antimicrobial drugs in some countries. The following practices have been clearly identified as contributing to the present situation:

- **Inappropriate prescribing of antibiotics;** e.g. for ailments for which they are ineffective, such as for sore throats where 80% of infective cases are caused by viruses (see Chapter 19).

- **Incorrect dose or duration of use;** e.g. in uncomplicated urinary tract infection more than 3 days of antibiotic treatment does not increase the chance of success, but does increase the risk of selection of resistance bacteria in the gut flora and adverse drug effects (see Chapter 20).

- **Excessive use of antibiotic prophylaxis;** e.g. for most types of surgery there is no value in giving more than one dose of antibiotic(s)

Part 3

General principles of usage of antimicrobial agents

Chapter 12

Use of the laboratory

This chapter covers the basic principles and limitations of using a micro-biology laboratory to obtain information on the selection and control of antimicrobial therapy. It is not a comprehensive account of the clinical laboratory microbiology. The examples used refer primarily to bacteriological practice, but the principles apply to the investigation of any infection.

In the diagnostic microbiology laboratory the aim is to identify the presence of pathogens as rapidly as possible and to provide, where applicable, antimicrobial susceptibility data to the clinician. A wide range of techniques, including microscopy, culture, antigen or antibody detection, and nucleic acid detection methods are used in the diagnostic laboratory. There is an increasing trend to standardize the protocols used to detect micro-organisms and their antimicrobial susceptibility. When using laboratory services, it is important to provide appropriate clinical details (e.g. travel history, antibiotic therapy) on the request form; without these the optimal use of diagnostic methods cannot be guaranteed. Clinical details may dictate the tests used and influence the interpretation of the result; e.g. in a patient treated with gentamicin (and a penicillin) for endocarditis the optimal serum aminoglycoside concentration is lower than that required in other infections. Crucially, many diagnostic methods, in particular those involving microbial culture are prone to biological variability, which may hinder the interpretation of results.

Specimen collection

Clinical laboratories rely on the quality of the specimens they receive; none more so than microbiology departments where the final result may depend on the degree of care observed in taking the specimen. A single contaminating bacterium introduced into a blood culture during collection may result in a patient being incorrectly diagnosed as having bacteraemia. Similarly, extraneous nucleic acid contaminating a sample can cause a false positive result, for example in mid-stream samples from women tested for chlamydial or gonococcal infection. Such an error could have profound consequences.

Some of the more common problems are listed.

- *Inappropriate specimen.* Saliva is submitted instead of sputum; a superficial skin swab is taken instead of a swab of pus (a specimen of pus in a sterile bottle is always preferable to a swab when possible).

- *Inadequate specimen.* The specimen may be too small (especially fluids for culture for tubercle bacilli). Rectal swabs are not an adequate substitute for faeces. It is almost impossible to interpret the significance of microbes cultured in tracheal aspirate in a patient who is ventilated, because of the likely presence of colonizing upper respiratory tract flora. Deep respiratory specimens, such as broncho-alveolar lavage fluid, are highly preferable to make an accurate diagnosis of pneumonia in such critically ill patients.

- *Wrong timing.* Specimens taken after the start of chemotherapy, when the causative organism may no longer be demonstrable, or after the patient has recovered. It is not uncommon for the laboratory to receive rock-hard faeces from patients with 'diarrhoea'. Many laboratories will not process non-diarrhoeal faecal samples.

- *Wrong container.* Blood for culture put in a plain (sometimes non-sterile) bottle instead of the correct culture fluid; biopsies put into bactericidal fixatives such as formalin.

- *Clerical errors.* Incorrect labelling; incomplete or misleading information on request forms.

Specimen transport

Prompt specimen transport to the laboratory is essential. Material submitted for culture may contain living cells; any delay in reaching the optimal cultural conditions will result in loss of viability. With fastidious organisms such as gonococci or viruses this may result in failure to isolate the organism. Conversely, overgrowth of pathogens by fast-growing commensals also commonly occurs during the period between collection of the specimen and processing in the laboratory, potentially obscuring true pathogens or resulting in a false positive result. For example, urine that is left at room temperature will act as a culture medium; bacteria that may be present in only low numbers may multiply to levels above the quantitative threshold that is used to define a positive result.

Specimens from potential medical emergencies, such as bacterial meningitis or malaria, should be delivered to the laboratory as soon as possible after

Table 12.2 Examples of a restricted range of antimicrobial agents selected for primary susceptibility testing of some common pathogens

Organism	Antimicrobial agents tested
Staphylococcus aureus	Benzylpenicillin
	Flucloxacillin (methicillin)
	Erythromycin
	Vancomycin
Streptococcus pyogenes (and other streptococci)	Benzylpenicillin
	Erythromycin
Anaerobes	Benzylpenicillin
	Clindamycin
	Metronidazole
Escherichia coli (and other enterobacteria)	Ampicillin (amoxicillin)
	Cephalosporins[a]
	Trimethoprim
	Ciprofloxacin
	Gentamicin
Pseudomonas aeruginosa	Piperacillin–tazobactam (ticarcillin–clavulanate)
	Gentamicin (tobramycin)
	Ciprofloxacin (ofloxacin)
	Meropenem (imipenem)
Urinary isolates	Ampicillin (amoxicillin)
	Cephradine or an alternative oral cephalosporin
	Trimethoprim
	Nalidixic acid (ciprofloxacin)
	Nitrofurantoin

[a] A representative of the earlier (e.g. cefradine, cefalexin) and later (e.g. cefuroxime, cefotaxime) cephalosporins, is usually chosen for primary testing. Agents shown in brackets are examples of acceptable alternatives.

antibacterial spectrum that only one representative of each needs to be tested. With other drugs where there is differential susceptibility of bacteria to different members of the group, such a decision is less easy. An organism susceptible to cefalexin, one of the earliest cephalosporins, is also usually susceptible to all subsequent members of that group and this is often used as a screen for cephalosporin-sensitive bacteria. However, the converse is not true; an organism resistant to cefalexin may be susceptible to later cephalosporins and a definitive statement in this regard can be made only by testing the appropriate compound. The same principle applies to nalidixic acid and newer, more active quinolones.

Interpreting antimicrobial susceptibility reports

Consider a report on pus from an abscess that grew *Staph. aureus*, which was resistant to penicillin, but susceptible to erythromycin and cloxacillin. The statement 'this organism is resistant to penicillin' means that penicillin would not influence the outcome. The infection may well improve due to host defences or to adequate drainage of pus, but since penicillin-resistant staphylococci are invariably β-lactamase producers any penicillin that reached the abscess would be rapidly destroyed. Such a statement is based on sound laboratory and clinical evidence. If the *Staph. aureus* isolate was found to have relatively low-level resistance (i.e. where inhibition of growth is incomplete but less than that produced using a susceptible control organism) the likelihood of clinical resistance to penicillin is more difficult to determine; factors such as site of infection and drug penetration may be important in this respect. The laboratory will try to weigh up the evidence and score the result as 'susceptible' or 'resistant'; the term 'reduced (or intermediate) susceptibility' is sometimes used, but this is a less satisfactory alternative and leaves the clinician uncertain how to interpret the result.

The statement 'this organism is susceptible to cloxacillin' implies that use of this antibiotic (or a related β-lactamase-stable penicillin) would influence the outcome. This is more difficult to support than a statement about resistance. Treatment with the antibiotic may elicit little response in the patient because insufficient drug may have penetrated into a large collection of pus; the dosage prescribed and route of administration may be important here. More importantly (although unlikely in the present example, since *Staph. aureus* is commonly incriminated in infected wounds) the wrong organism (an innocent bystander) may have been tested. Host factors that may also influence therapeutic outcome are described in Chapter 13.

Conclusion

When in doubt, whether about the optimal specimen to submit, the interpretation of a test result or the most appropriate treatment, the laboratory should be consulted. For unusual diseases and problem cases it is often possible to seek help from specialized units such as tropical hospitals and institutes. In some countries reference laboratories are available that provide expertise in particular areas. In the UK many of these operate under the aegis of the Health Protection Agency at Colindale. Worldwide, the Centers for Disease Control and Prevention, Atlanta, Georgia, USA, offer a service for the diagnosis and therapy of unusual infectious diseases.

Further reading

Fawley WN, Wilcox MH. Molecular diagnostic techniques. *Medicine* 2005; **33**: 26–32.

Yang S, Rothman RE. PCR-based diagnostics for infectious diseases: uses, limitations, and future applications in acute-care settings. *Lancet Infectious Diseases* 2004; **4**: 337–348.

Chapter 13

General principles of the treatment of infection

Antimicrobial agents are among the most commonly prescribed drugs. Their use has had a major impact on the control of most bacterial infections in man and to a lesser, although constantly increasing, degree, is affecting the outcome of many fungal, viral, protozoal, and helminthic infections. However, there are concerns that unnecessary use is compromising their beneficial effect. The principles governing the use of antimicrobial agents to be discussed in this chapter apply specifically to the management of bacterial infections, although the overall approach is similar when selecting treatment for other microbial diseases.

Antimicrobial therapy demands an initial clinical evaluation of the nature and extent of the infective process and knowledge of the likely causative pathogen(s). This assessment should be supported, whenever practicable, by laboratory investigation aimed at establishing the microbial aetiology and its susceptibility to antimicrobial agents appropriate for the treatment of the infection. The choice of drug, its dose, route, and frequency of administration are also dependent upon an appreciation of the pharmacological and pharmacokinetic features of a particular agent. Furthermore, the range and predictability of adverse reactions of a particular compound should be kept in mind.

Clinical assessment

The clinical evaluation should define the anatomical location and severity of the infective process. The history and examination frequently determine such infective states as meningitis, arthritis, pneumonia, and cellulitis. Although such diseases may be caused by a wide variety of organisms, the range of pathogens is usually limited, and the pattern of susceptibility reasonably predictable. This, therefore, permits a rational selection of chemotherapy in the initial management of such infections.

The anatomical location is not only critical from the point of view of the most likely pathogen and the most suitable choice of drug, but also determines the route of administration. Superficial infections of the skin, such as impetigo, which is caused by *Streptococcus pyogenes*, or infection of the mucous membranes such as oral or vaginal candidiasis, caused by *Candida albicans*, respond well to topical application. However, if infection is caused by the microbial invasion of tissues or the bloodstream, adequate tissue concentrations of a drug may be achieved only by intravenous or intramuscular administration.

Other clues as to the nature of the infection are gleaned from epidemiological considerations such as the age, sex, and occupation of the patient. In tropical countries, diseases such as malaria, amoebiasis, and salmonellosis (including typhoid fever) are prime suspects in the investigation of fever and diarrhoea, and local knowledge about the prevalence of diseases such as filariasis, schistosomiasis, and trypanosomiasis, which are circumscribed in distribution, may be used to advantage. In countries free from these diseases as indigenous problems, a history of overseas travel should alert the physician to consider exotic infections.

Pre-existing medical problems may predispose to infection; such conditions include valvular heart disease, underlying malignant disease, or the presence of prosthetic devices such as artificial hip joints, heart valves, or intravascular cannulae.

Under some circumstances the invading pathogen may be part of the host's normal flora. The normal host defences may be breached in a variety of ways. For example, the skin or mucous membranes, which are normally a most effective barrier against infection, may permit access of pathogenic organisms to the deeper tissues when traumatized by a surgical incision or by accident. Similarly, burns can denude large areas of the body with subsequent infection by bacteria, notably *Pseudomonas aeruginosa*, *Staphylococcus aureus*, and *Str. pyogenes*, which may be acquired from contact with patients or staff within the hospital.

The circulating and tissue phagocytes, together with the complement system and antibodies, provide an important defence against infection. Therefore, an absolute or relative deficiency of circulating polymorphonuclear leucocytes is commonly associated with recurrent, frequently serious, infection. In patients with acute leukaemia, cytotoxic chemotherapy often depresses the circulating leucocytes to low levels for several days or weeks. Such patients are extremely vulnerable to serious episodes of infection, particularly bloodstream invasion, which carries a high mortality if untreated.

Laboratory assessment

Few infective conditions present such a typical picture that a definitive clinical and microbiological diagnosis can be made without recourse to the laboratory. Therefore, whenever possible, a clinical diagnosis should be supported by laboratory confirmation. Such confirmation makes both the diagnosis and the management, in particular the selection of antimicrobial chemotherapy, more certain and allows for a more sound assessment of the likely prognosis. However, when infection is obvious or strongly suspected on clinical grounds, therapy should be instituted as soon as appropriate specimens for laboratory investigation have been taken. In some cases (e.g. pneumococcal or meningococcal meningitis) the patient's chances of survival are directly related to the promptness with which therapy is started. Furthermore, laboratory reports are not always contributory and several days may be lost trying to establish a microbiological diagnosis, during which time the patient's condition may deteriorate.

Serological tests that demonstrate antibody against specific microbial antigens are important in the diagnosis of more persistent infections such as syphilis, brucellosis, and Q fever. Tests to demonstrate the presence of microbial antigens are also valuable in the diagnosis of selected infections. For example, fluorescent antibody reagents can detect *Pneumocystis carinii* (jiroveci) in sputum or bronchial lavage material, and pneumococcal antigen is often present in the urine of patients with pneumococcal pneumonia.

Assessment of sepsis and the systemic inflammatory response

Sepsis is defined as the combination of symptoms or signs of a localized primary site of infection plus a systemic inflammatory response. The presence of systemic inflammatory response is often the first sign that infection is spreading from the primary site and that the patient may be bacteraemic (see Chapter 22). The systemic inflammatory response syndrome is defined by the presence of two or more of the following indicators:

* temperature $>38°C$ or $<36°C$
* heart rate >90 beats/min
* respiratory rate >20 breaths/min or alveolar pressure of carbon dioxide ($PaCO_2$) <4.3 kPa
* peripheral white blood cell count (WBC) $>12\,000$ cells/mm^3 or <4000 cells/mm^3

Infection is not the only cause of systemic inflammatory response syndrome. Other common causes include: accidental or elective trauma (it is a normal reaction to elective surgery); chronic inflammatory conditions (e.g. arteritis, systemic lupus erythematosus); and malignancy (especially lymphoma but also solid tumours). Also, the syndrome can be a response to infection by any type of pathogen, bacterial, fungal, protozoal, and viral. None the less measurement of inflammatory response is a key part of the clinical assessment of bacterial infection. For example, if a woman presenting with dysuria plus frequency is found to have the systemic inflammatory response syndrome it means that she is unlikely to have simple cystitis (Chapter 20), but that infection has spread into the kidney and possibly into the bloodstream.

Severe sepsis is defined as sepsis plus evidence of organ dysfunction, hypoperfusion or hypotension. Evidence of perfusion abnormalities affecting the vital organs (brain, heart, kidneys, lungs) includes acute confusion, hypotension, oliguria, and hypoxia or lactic acidosis.

Septic shock is defined as sepsis with hypotension that persists despite adequate fluid resuscitation, along with the presence of perfusion abnormalities.

The importance of this classification of the severity of systemic infection is clear from considering 30-day mortality associated with bacteraemia. On average this is 10–20%, but increases to 20–30% with systemic inflammatory response syndrome, 30–50% with severe sepsis and 50–80% with septic shock.

Selection of antimicrobial chemotherapy

In-vitro susceptibility

In-vitro testing of drugs provides indirect evidence of the likely clinical response of a particular pathogen to a specific drug or drugs. Confirmation of clinical efficacy can be determined only in vivo; hence the importance of clinical evaluation of all new antimicrobial agents. Controlled experimental evidence gained from the treatment of artificial infections in animals provides only indirect evidence of the likely clinical efficacy. Occasionally in-vitro evidence of activity is not borne out by in-vivo evidence of success. For example, *Salmonella enterica* serotype Typhi is susceptible in vitro to many drugs active against Gram-negative bacilli, including gentamicin; however, typhoid fever responds clinically only to a limited range of drugs, including ciprofloxacin, ceftriaxone, chloramphenicol, amoxicillin, and co-trimoxazole. This may in part be due to the intracellular location of the pathogen in this disease.

Bacteristatic or bactericidal agents

Antibacterial agents are often separated into either bactericidal or bacteristatic agents according to their ability to kill or inhibit bacterial growth.

Examples of bactericidal drugs include the β-lactam agents and fluoroquinolones; bacteristatic agents include the tetracyclines and chloramphenicol. This separation is somewhat artificial since some bacteristatic drugs may be bactericidal either in higher concentrations or against different bacterial species. Bacteristatic agents must rely on host defences, in particular the phagocytic cells, to finally eliminate the infection, since if the drug is withdrawn bacteria have the opportunity to recover. Under most circumstances the choice between a bactericidal or a bacteristatic agent is not critical. This is not the case in the treatment of infective endocarditis. Here bacteria are protected against phagocytic activity within the vegetations present on the deformed or prosthetic heart valve or adjacent endocardium. Under these circumstances it is important to use a bactericidal drug or combination of drugs that penetrate the vegetations and thus eradicate the infection. Similarly, patients with neutropenia from cytotoxic chemotherapy or other causes of bone marrow aplasia are extremely vulnerable to infection. Bacteristatic drugs are inappropriate in these cases and bactericidal agents should be selected.

Pharmacokinetic factors

The aim of chemotherapy is to eliminate an infection as rapidly as possible. To achieve this a sufficient concentration of the drug or drugs selected must reach the site of infection. The choice of agent is, therefore, as much dependent upon the pharmacological and pharmacokinetic features of the drugs, which determine absorption, distribution, metabolism, and excretion, as upon its antimicrobial properties. These aspects are discussed in more detail in Chapter 14.

In general, drugs are administered either topically, by mouth, or by intravenous or intramuscular injection. Oral absorption is most erratic. Drugs must first negotiate the acid condition of the stomach before being absorbed, usually from the proximal small bowel. This occurs most readily when the stomach is empty and it is generally advised that they be swallowed approximately 30 min before or 4 h after a meal.

Absorption can be increased by protecting a drug from acid inactivation by a coating (so-called enteric coating), which subsequently breaks down once the tablet is beyond the stomach. Alternatively, the drug may be modified chemically to produce a more acid-stable formulation (see p. 198). For most minor infections, including skin, soft-tissue, respiratory tract, and lower urinary tract infection, oral therapy is appropriate.

In contrast to oral administration, intravenous administration avoids the vagaries of gastrointestinal absorption, and achieves rapid therapeutic blood and tissue concentrations. Intramuscular administration requires absorption through the tissue capillaries and is generally rapid except in conditions of cardiovascular collapse and shock, when tissue perfusion is impaired. Relatively avascular sites such as the aqueous, and in particular the vitreous humour of the eye, are difficult sites in which to achieve adequate concentrations of drugs. In contrast, the presence of inflammation increases the permeability of many natural barriers such as the meninges and in this situation allows higher concentrations of certain drugs, such as the penicillins, to be achieved within the cerebrospinal fluid. Other drugs, most notably chloramphenicol, are little influenced by such inflammatory changes.

Choice of antimicrobial regimens

Drug dosing

There are no universally applicable guidelines for drug dosing. However, awareness of the relationship between the pharmacokinetic profile of a drug and the minimum inhibitory concentration (MIC) against a target pathogen has greatly assisted in better defining dosage regimens of some antibiotics. These provide a pharmacodynamic prediction of the optimum dosage regimen. Other factors that influence drug dosing are tolerability and toxicity. Some agents, most notably the penicillins, have such a wide margin of safety that high doses are frequently prescribed. Only in a few cases (e.g. treatment of *Ps. aeruginosa* infection with ticarcillin) does such antimicrobial overkill have a microbiologically rational basis. The ratio of peak plasma concentration (C_{max}) to the MIC, or area under the curve (AUC) to MIC (Fig. 13.1) is often used to calculate the dose and frequency of administration to ensure the most effective drug concentrations. The C_{max}:MIC ratio is the best predictor of bacterial killing for the aminoglycosides and quinolones, while

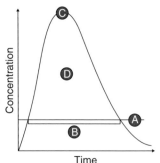

Fig. 13.1 Relationship between the pharmacokinetic profile of an antibiotic and the minimum inhibitory concentration against a hypothetical target micro-organism. (A) Minimum inhibitory concentration; (B) time above minimum inhibitory concentration; (C) peak; (D) area under the curve > minimum inhibitory concentration. Redrawn from: Finch RG. Antimicrobial therapy: principles of use. *Medicine* 2005; **33**: 42–46 with permission from Lippincott, Williams & Wilkins.

the AUC:MIC ratio is used to determine dosage schedules for β-lactam agents. In the case of bacterial meningitis much higher ratios are required to achieve therapeutic concentrations in the cerebrospinal fluid. However, for many licensed agents, the dosages are based on experience gained from clinical trials of the treatment of a wide variety of infections and are included in the *Summary of Product Characteristics* Data Sheets for approved agents.

Length of therapy

Treatment should continue until all micro-organisms are eliminated from the tissues or the infection has been sufficiently controlled for the normal host defences to eradicate it. This end-point is in general determined by clinical observation and evidence of the resolution of the inflammatory process such as the return of body temperature and white cell count to normal. Microbiological end-points may be appropriate for some infections, such as urinary tract infections where repeat urine cultures can be obtained 1 week and 4 weeks after stopping therapy. These will indicate failed treatment and recurrent infection respectively. However, other outcomes include length of stay and time to discharge (for those in hospital), and time to return to former activities. These factors are important when determining the health economics of disease management.

Many infections come under control within a few days and 5–7 days' treatment is often sufficient. Uncomplicated urinary tract infections usually respond very rapidly to chemotherapy. Selection of the least dose compatible with complete resolution is desirable (see Chapter 20). In contrast, patients with pulmonary tuberculosis require 6 months' treatment with isoniazid and rifampicin if relapse is to be prevented (see Chapter 25). Furthermore, 10 days' penicillin treatment is necessary to eradicate *Str. pyogenes* from the throat in patients with streptococcal tonsillitis, although symptomatic improvement occurs within a few days. There is no universally 'correct' duration of chemotherapy and each problem should be judged on its merits based on the clinical response to treatment.

Adverse reactions

Antimicrobial agents, like all other therapeutic substances, have the potential to produce adverse reactions. These vary widely in their nature, frequency, and severity. Many reactions, such as gastrointestinal intolerance, are minor and short lived but others may be serious, life-threatening, and occasionally fatal. Drug reactions are unfortunately a common cause of prolonged stay in hospital or may precipitate hospital admission. Drug reactions may be predictable and dose dependent, for example nephrotoxicity associated with the use of the antifungal agent amphotericin B. However, many adverse reactions are unpredictable. The subject is discussed more fully in Chapter 16.

Combined therapy

In general, single-drug therapy of established infections is preferred, whenever possible. Such an approach is known to be effective and reduces the risks of adverse reactions and drug interactions that may accompany multiple-drug prescribing, as well as the cost of treatment. None the less, there are a few situations in which combined chemotherapy has definite advantages over single drug therapy.

Initial therapy

In the management of acute and potentially life-threatening infections, combined chemotherapy covering all likely pathogens is often used until the cause of the infection is established. It is common practice to combine flucloxacillin with an aminoglycoside, such as gentamicin, in the initial treatment of serious infections. However, should there be evidence that the infection has arisen in association with mucosal surfaces, such as the gut or female genital tract, then metronidazole is frequently added to meet the possibility of a mixed anaerobic and aerobic bacterial infection. Once a definitive diagnosis is established it is important to adjust the therapeutic regimen to one that is most appropriate.

Synergy

Under some circumstances combined chemotherapy is selected for its known synergic effect on a pathogenic organism. This increased ability to inhibit or kill the pathogen may speed resolution or reduce the risk of relapse when treating difficult infections. One of the commonest requirements for synergic therapy is the treatment of infective endocarditis caused by enterococci and occasionally by oral streptococci. The combination of two bactericidal drugs, penicillin and gentamicin (or streptomycin), is synergic both in vitro and in vivo and is associated with a more favourable response to treatment than is single-drug therapy.

Antagonism

Some drugs may have an opposite effect and be antagonistic. For example, shortly after penicillin and tetracycline became available, it was shown that the two drugs together produced a worse clinical result in the treatment

Chapter 14

Pharmacokinetics

Ehrlich's 'magic bullet' notion of chemotherapy foresaw substances that when given as a single dose would localize in the sites of infection and destroy the organisms there. Despite the enormous advances made in the development of antimicrobial compounds, none exhibits the remarkable properties Ehrlich visualized. Most antimicrobial agents are widely distributed in the body in response to forces that have nothing to do with infection and may result in concentrations of the agent being least in the sites where they are most needed.

Basis for therapeutic action

Among the many properties that must be exhibited by therapeutically useful chemotherapeutic agents, the ability to achieve effective concentrations and act in the complex environment of the infected lesion is essential. When antibiotics are given systemically the delivery and maintenance of effective concentrations at the site of infection are determined by the concentrations achieved in the blood, which are in turn determined by the absorption, distribution, metabolism, and elimination of the drug, and by the way in which the blood-borne drug is distributed to the tissues. From serial measurements of the concentration of the agent in the serum—usually in healthy volunteers—it is possible to calculate both its rates of absorption and elimination and the volume in which the drug is distributed. The volume of distribution indicates whether it is largely confined within the vascular compartment or spreads out into the extracellular fluid—the site of most infections—or penetrates into cells where some organisms, for example mycobacteria and brucellae, multiply. The rates of transfer, volume of distribution, and other key properties can be given numerical values that provide succinct and quantitative statements of the drug pharmacokinetics. In this respect antimicrobials do not differ from other drugs. However, in comparison with other drugs, information about intestinal elimination and distribution into tissues has special relevance for antimicrobial agents. Intestinal elimination determines the amount of an antimicrobial drug that reaches the colon, the impact on the normal flora there and therefore the risk of adverse effects such as *Clostridium difficile* colitis. Infections can occur in any tissue in the body and some pathogens survive within mammalian cells; therefore, unlike other drugs the anatomical location of target receptors for antimicrobials is highly variable.

Plasma half-life

The time required for the concentration of drug in the plasma to fall by half is called the plasma half-life. Half-lives of different antibiotics vary considerably. That of benzylpenicillin, for example, is only 30 min, whereas that of the antimalarial mefloquine is about 3 weeks.

The concentration achieved in plasma while the drug is resident in the body can be measured relatively simply, but the calculation of the true half-life must take into account the distribution phase (sometimes called α-phase) during which the compound is migrating from the plasma to the tissues; this is clearly influenced by the route of administration, since absorption from intestinal or intramuscular sites is not instantaneous (Fig. 14.1).

The half-life of a drug that is usually cited is that which follows distribution to the tissues and is designated the β-phase. Any metabolism of the drug, binding to plasma proteins, or alteration in the functional integrity of the organs of excretion (usually the kidney or the liver, or both) will affect the elimination of the drug and hence the plasma half-life.

Drug accumulation

If large doses are given or the half-life of the drug is such that complete elimination has not occurred before the next dose is administered, the concentration of drug in the plasma will progressively rise. The excretion phase being logarithmic, the rate of elimination rises as the concentration of drug rises; eventually excretion proceeds as fast as the accumulation and the drug reaches a steady state (Fig. 14.2). In this example the first dose results in plasma concentration that exceeds the minimum inhibitory concentration for the organism being treated but not throughout the dosing interval. If it is essential to reach higher concentrations immediately then a loading dose should be given, which is usually two to three times the maintenance dose.

The possibility of accumulation and its consequences must be considered when an agent with a long half-life is administered or the patient's capacity to eliminate the agent is known or thought likely to be impaired and the agent has dose-related side effects.

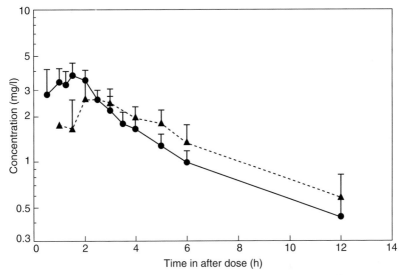

Fig. 14.1 Mean plasma (●) and inflammatory fluid (▲) concentrations following a single 750-mg oral dose of ciprofloxacin. The distribution (or α) phase lasts for 2 h and is followed by the elimination (or β) phase. There is an even longer distribution phase in the inflammatory fluid where concentrations do not peak until about 3 h after administration. There is a lag in diffusion of drug back into the plasma so that from 3 h after administration tissue fluid concentrations are higher than plasma concentrations. Reproduced from C. Catchpole, J.M. Andrews, J. Woodcock, and R. Wise. The comparative pharmacokinetics and tissue penetration of single-dose ciprofloxacin 400mg i.v. and 750 mg po. J. Antimicrob Chemother 33(1): 103–110, 1994 by permission of Oxford University Press.

Absorption

Many antibiotics do not produce adequate plasma levels when given by mouth and are available only as injectable preparations. In some countries injections are favoured over oral therapy, but this has more to do with cultural differences and traditions than with proven therapeutic benefit. In the UK antibiotics are usually given by mouth whenever possible, particularly in domiciliary practice, because of the convenience of the oral route. The need for properties such as stability in solution means that pharmaceutical preparations (injections, capsules, tablets, syrups, etc.) can contain different derivatives of the drug, sometimes with distinct properties.

Oral administration

The fraction of a dose of an oral drug that is absorbed unchanged and available to interact with the target is known as its bioavailability. The degree

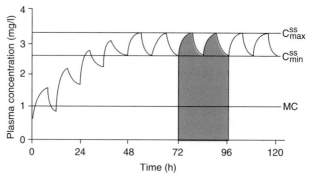

Fig. 14.2 Illustration of a drug dosed twice daily that takes five doses to reach steady state. The shaded area shows the area under the concentration-time curve at steady state over 24 h. C_{max}^{ss} is the maximum (or peak) concentration at steady state and C_{min}^{ss} is the minimum (or trough) concentration at steady state. MIC is the minimum inhibitory concentration for a target pathogen. Reproduced from 'Basis of Anti-Infective Therapy: Pharmacokinetic - Pharmacodynamic Criteria and Methodology for Dual Dosage Individualisation' by A. Sanchez-Navarro and MM Sanchez Recio, *Clinical Pharmacokinetics*; 1999, **37**(4): 289–304, with permission from Wolters Kluwer Health.

to which antimicrobial compounds are absorbed when given orally differs greatly (Table 14.1). Absorption is one factor that determines the effect that an antimicrobial has on the normal flora of the colon but intestinal elimination is also important.

Antibiotic esters (pro-drugs)

Some drugs that can be given orally are nevertheless irregularly absorbed and often produce low plasma concentrations. Erythromycin is one example of this, and several derivatives have been produced in an attempt to overcome the difficulty, including erythromycin estolate, which is microbiologically inactive, but is much more lipid soluble than the parent drug and much better absorbed in the small intestine, where non-specific esterases liberate the active erythromycin into the portal vein. Esterification as the means of improving the oral absorption of drugs has been fairly widely used, other examples being the esters of ampicillin, such as pivampicillin, and aciclovir (valaciclovir). Such microbiologically inactive compounds that are converted to the active form are known as pro-drugs.

Esters such as cefuroxime axetil allow drugs that must otherwise be administered by injection to be given orally. Others, like the erythromycin and ampicillin esters, increase the poor absorption of the native compound.

of 25–40 litres, intracellular distribution is implied. In rare circumstances, distribution volumes may be measured in hundreds or even thousands of litres. These large volumes suggest extensive binding to intracellular protein or organelles.

Drug concentrations in tissue biopsies

Drug concentrations are measures in homogenized tissue samples; the result is therefore an average of the extracellular and intracellular concentrations. However, because cells make up about 70% of the volume of most tissue samples the intracellular concentration has a dominant influence so that the result is not a good indicator of drug concentration in extracellular fluid, which is where most pathogens are located. For example, β-lactam antibiotics do not penetrate eukaryotic cells. Suppose that the concentration of a β-lactam in extracellular fluid is 10 mg/l: the concentration in a homogenized tissue biopsy would be only 3 mg/l because extracellular fluid accounts for only 30% of the biopsy.

Most intracellular bacterial infections occur in the lung where distribution of antibacterial drugs has been relatively well characterized. This information is of direct relevance to the management of infections caused by the obligate intracellular pathogens that cause pneumonia (*Legionella pneumophila, Chlamydophila pneumoniae, Mycobacterium tuberculosis*). Ability to penetrate eukaryotic cells is a prerequisite for drugs aimed at infections caused by these organisms. However, high lung tissue concentrations are of less certain relevance in most lung infections, which are caused by extracellular pathogens.

Metabolism

Many antibiotics are modified in the body; the resulting metabolites are important for several reasons. First, they are generally, though not always, microbiologically less active than the parent compound. Some metabolites show not only different degrees, but also different spectra, of activity. In addition, metabolites may differ from the parent compounds in toxicity. If they are relatively inactive and more toxic, conventional microbiological assay of the drug will give very poor guidance as to the toxic hazard. This is particularly true of allergy, which can be triggered by tiny concentrations of minor metabolites rather than the parent compound. Finally, the metabolites may display altered pharmacokinetic characteristics, so that the period for which they are present in the body and able to achieve an antibacterial (or toxic) effect may be longer, or shorter than that of the parent compound.

Occasionally, it is necessary to prevent metabolism from occurring. The carbapenem antibiotic imipenem is susceptible to a renal dehydropeptidase that opens the β-lactam ring. Consequently, imipenem is formulated with a dehydropeptidase inhibitor, cilastatin, which protects it from inactivation.

Antimicrobial agents that are metabolized are particularly liable to interact with other drugs. This is most likely to be a problem in intensive care, where patients are critically ill and receiving multiple drugs. Antimicrobial compounds that inhibit the metabolism of other drugs in the liver include macrolides, fluoroquinolones, and antifungal azoles. On the other hand, rifampicin is a non-specific inducer of hepatic metabolism and may therefore cause therapeutic failure of other co-administered drugs by increasing their clearance. Drugs frequently used in intensive care that are at risk of clinically relevant pharmacokinetic interactions with anti-infective agents include some benzodiazepines (especially midazolam and triazolam), immunosuppressive agents (cyclosporin, tacrolimus), anti-asthmatic agents (theophylline), opioid analgesics (alfentanil), anticonvulsants (phenytoin, carbamazepine), calcium antagonists (verapamil, nifedipine, felodipine), and anticoagulants (warfarin).

Elimination

Intestinal elimination

The human body harbours a large number of bacteria that have important functions, particularly in the gut. The adverse effects of antibiotics on the normal flora include emergence of resistant strains from among the normal flora and replacement of the normal flora by more harmful organisms, such as pathogenic fungi or *Clostridium difficile*. Bioavailability of commonly prescribed antimicrobial drugs varies quite widely (Table 14.1). In general, poorly absorbed oral compounds have a more profound effect on the normal flora of the colon. However, after absorption from the gut drugs may be eliminated from the body by secretion into bile or by secretion by enterocytes. Thus even intravenously administered antimicrobial agents may reach the gut in sufficient quantities to cause harmful effects on the normal flora.

Renal elimination

Most antibiotics are eliminated by the kidneys, so that very high concentrations may be achieved in urine. Excretion is by glomerular filtration or tubular secretion, and sometimes both. The principal compounds excreted in the urine by active tubular secretion are the penicillins and cephalosporins. This process is so effective as to clear the blood of most of the drug during its passage through the kidney, and these compounds generally have a very short half-life of 2 h or less. Increasing the frequency of administration can increase the period for which inhibitory levels of rapidly excreted agents are present in the blood. Alternatively, an agent that competes for the active transport mechanism may be used. The oral uricosuric agent probenecid shares the tubular route of excretion of penicillins and can be used to prolong the plasma half-life of these antibiotics.

Influence of infection

The vast majority of information about the pharmacokinetics of antimicrobial drugs comes from studies in normal volunteers. Infection is likely to change absorption, distribution, and elimination so plasma concentrations in patients may be profoundly different from those found in normal volunteers (Fig. 14.3).

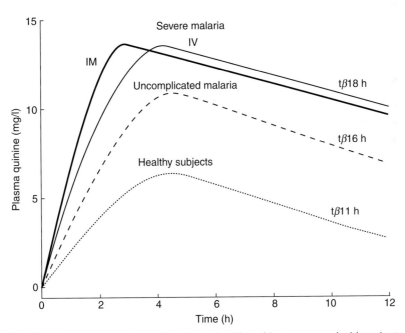

Fig. 14.3 Plasma concentrations of quinine in healthy subjects compared with patients with uncomplicated and severe malaria following administration of a loading dose of 20 mg (salt)/kg. Reproduced from J.White. Antimalarial pharmacokinetics and treatment regimens. *British Journal of Clinical Pharmacology* 1992; **34**: 1–10 with permission from Blackwell Publishing.

Pharmacodynamics

In contrast to pharmacokinetics, which describes the way a drug is handled in the body, pharmacodynamics specifies the way the drug interacts with the microbial target in the conditions imposed by pharmacokinetic fluctuations. This aspect of drug action is much more speculative, since it is not normally susceptible to direct measurement in situ, but is valuable insofar as it tries to define the dosing pattern likely to lead to the most efficient eradication of the offending microbe.

Among the factors to be considered are: whether the area under the concentration–time curve is more important than the peak level achieved; whether the regular replenishment of an inhibitory concentration for a short period is more, or less, efficacious than a continuously maintained inhibitory level; and whether antimicrobial activity is prolonged beyond the time for which an inhibitory concentration is achieved—the so-called post-antibiotic effect (p. 31).

Such judgements rely heavily on knowledge of how the micro-organism responds in laboratory controlled conditions in vitro and models of varying degrees of elaboration are sometimes constructed to try to approximate more closely to the dynamic circumstances that exist in life. Extrapolation of these observations to the in-vivo situation depends on the assumption that similar behaviour can be expected to occur in the complex, fluctuating conditions within an infected lesion and, indeed, on whether concentrations at the site of infection can be reliably predicted given individual variation.

Perhaps the most extraordinary feature of antimicrobial pharmacokinetics is that, after more than 50 years of intensive clinical and experimental study, the shape of drug concentration–time curve that is needed at the site of infection to secure optimum antimicrobial effects is still not known. If we knew that, we would be one step (of several required) towards more rationally based dosage schedules.

Further reading

Barger A, Fuhst C, Wiedemann B. Pharmacological indices in antibiotic therapy. *Journal of Antimicrobial Chemotherapy* 2003; **52**: 893–898.

Craig WA. Pharmacokinetic/pharmacodynamic parameters: rationale for antibacterial dosing of mice and men. *Clinical Infectious Diseases* 1998; **26**: 1–10.

Pea F, Furlanut M. Pharmacokinetic aspects of treating infections in the intensive care unit: focus on drug interactions. *Clinical Pharmacokinetics* 2001; **40**: 833–868.

Table 16.1 (continued) Relative frequency of selected adverse reactions to antimicrobial agents (The more serious or important adverse drug reactions are shown in bold type). Reproduced by Davey P., 'Antimicrobial Chemotherapy' in DJ Weatherall, JGG Ledingham, and DA Warrell (eds.) *Oxford Textbook of Medicine*, Third edn., Vol. 1 (1996), with permission from Oxford University Press.

Antimicrobial agent	Frequent	Infrequent
Rifampicin	Hepatotoxicity	Hypersensitivity
	Liver enzyme induction	'Influenza syndrome' (intermittent treatment)
		Haematological toxicity
Tetracyclines	Gastrointestinal intolerance	Photosensitivity
	Candidiasis	Nephrotoxicity
	Dental staining and hypoplasia in childhood	
Vancomycin	'Red man' syndrome	**Nephrotoxicity**

Chemical

Many intravenously administered drugs, including antimicrobial agents, produce local irritation and frank phlebitis. To overcome this it may be necessary to adjust the pH of an intravenous infusion by suitable buffering. Similarly, pain may accompany the intramuscular injection of a drug. For example, cefoxitin is given with a local anaesthetic, lignocaine, to counter the pain at the injection site.

Many drugs may produce gastrointestinal symptoms due to a local chemical irritation of the gastric and intestinal mucosa. Here again, suitable buffering, enteric coating, or slow-release formulations may diminish these symptoms and increase the acceptability of a drug.

Metabolic

Drug accumulation

Drugs usually undergo oxidation, reduction, hydrolysis, or conjugation to a greater or lesser degree before excretion. The liver is the major site of this metabolism, although other organs such as the kidneys are also involved. When disease impairs renal or hepatic function there is the risk of accumulation of the drug, or a metabolite, which may reach toxic concentrations in the tissues.

Similarly, in the premature or full-term neonate both renal and hepatic functions are physiologically immature so that some adjustments of dosaging may have to be made (see Chapter 15).

Enzyme induction

Certain drugs may cause hepatic enzyme induction or the synthesis of a new enzyme. Rifampicin is a powerful inducer, decreasing the half-lives of many drugs such as prednisone, warfarin, digoxin, ketoconazole, and the sulphonylureas. Women simultaneously prescribed rifampicin and the contraceptive pill may conceive owing to inadequate circulating hormone concentrations that result from the induction of hepatic enzymes by rifampicin. Likewise, simultaneous administration of certain quinolones (e.g. ciprofloxacin) may result in the accumulation of toxic concentrations of theophyllines.

Electrolyte overload

Certain antibiotics such as piperacillin and ticarcillin, being relatively inactive, are prescribed in large doses. Each 1 g of these agents contains 4.7 mmol sodium. This can result in sodium overloading and congestive cardiac failure, particularly in patients with impaired renal function.

Dental staining

Tetracyclines are taken up by developing bones and teeth. In the former this causes no significant long-term complications, but staining of the teeth is unsightly and ranges from patchy cream to extensive brown deposits. Enamel hypoplasia may also result. The ability to cause dental staining varies among the tetracyclines, being least with oxytetracycline. However, avoidance of all tetracyclines in children under 12 years of age will prevent staining of the permanent dentition.

Histamine release

Too-rapid infusion of vancomycin can result in the release of histamine, which in turn, can produce acute flushing, tachycardia, and hypotension—a reaction descriptively known as 'red man' syndrome.

Drug interactions

Drugs may interact with other agents in vitro when mixed before administration, or in vivo once the drugs are ingested or injected. The study of drug interactions has become increasingly important and complex as new therapeutic agents become available. In general, incompatibilities can be avoided by mixing the agents separately and administering them by a different route or at different times.

Table 16.2 In-vitro incompatibilities of selected antimicrobial agents

Antimicrobial agent	Agents with which incompatibility exists
Penicillin G	Metronidazole, tetracyclines, vancomycin, amphotericin B
Flucloxacillin	Blood products; aminoglycosides if mixed
Cefuroxime	Aminoglycosides if mixed
Clindamycin	Ampicillin, phenytoin, ranitidine
Vancomycin	Hydrocortisone, heparin
Gentamicin	Penicillins, cephalosporins, erythromycin, heparin

In-vitro incompatibilities

Table 16.2 indicates the variety of in-vitro incompatibilities associated with antimicrobial agents. This list is far from complete. Pharmaceutical advice should be sought or the relevant section of the *British National Formulary* consulted whenever there is doubt.

In-vivo interactions

In-vivo drug interactions include competition for plasma protein-binding sites and inhibition or induction of liver enzymes, thus interfering with or potentiating other therapeutic effects. Table 16.3 indicates the variety of effects that have been described. Among the more important is interference with anticoagulant drugs, a problem that is commonly, but not exclusively, caused by antimicrobial agents. For example, rifampicin and griseofulvin impair anticoagulation by enzyme induction, whereas sulphonamides, co-trimoxazole, erythromycin, metronidazole, and the azole antifungals increase anticoagulation by enzyme inhibition, so that bleeding may occur.

Hypersensitivity

Among the antibiotics the β-lactam compounds have the greatest potential to produce hypersensitivity reactions. Because of the similar structure of the penicillins, hypersensitivity to one agent is usually accompanied by hypersensitivity to the whole group. Moreover, structural similarities between cephalosporins and penicillins are accompanied by a degree of cross-hypersensitivity: about 10% of patients who are hypersensitive to penicillins show cross-hypersensitivity to cephalosporins. This is much more likely to occur in patients who have experienced a previous anaphylactic response to a penicillin, when the subsequent use of all β-lactam antibiotics (see

Table 16.3 In-vivo incompatibilities of selected antimicrobial agents

Antibiotic(s)	Interacting agent(s)	Adverse reaction
Aminoglycosides	Non-depolarizing muscle relaxants	Neuromuscular blockade
Chloramphenicol Metronidazole Isoniazid	Phenytoin	Phenytoin toxicity
Ciprofloxacin Clarithromycin Erythromycin	Theophylline	Agitation, convulsions
Fluconazole	Warfarin	Increased anticoagulation
Griseofulvin	Warfarin	Decreased anticoagulation
Itraconazole Ketoconazole	Oral antacids and H_2 antagonists	Decreased absorption of antifungals
Aminoglycosides Ketoconazole Quinolones	Cyclosporin A	Cyclosporin nephrotoxicity
Metronidazole	Alcohol	Nausea and vomiting (disulfiram effect)
Rifampicin	Oral contraceptives	Decreased contraceptive efficacy
Co-trimoxazole Sulphonamides	Anticoagulants	Increased anticoagulation
Tetracyclines	Oral antacid preparations and oral iron	Decreased tetracycline absorption

Chapter 1) must be avoided. The monobactam agent aztreonam is less allergenic and may be given to patients with a history of hypersensitivity to other β-lactam antibiotics. This suggests that the β-lactam ring is not the sensitizing moiety of these drugs.

Immediate reactions

Immediate hypersensitivity reactions to penicillins and cephalosporins can, within minutes, produce nausea, vomiting, pruritus, urticaria, wheezing, laryngeal oedema, and cardiovascular collapse. In extreme cases the patient may die unless the attack is controlled with adrenaline and attention to the integrity of the airways. The estimated frequency for anaphylaxis is 1–5 for every 10 000 courses of penicillin prescribed.

The nucleoside analogues used in the treatment of HIV disease are all associated with peripheral neuropathy.

Neuromuscular blockade, although rare, is potentially serious and occurs in association with the use of aminoglycosides and tetracyclines. The aminoglycosides produce neuromuscular blockade by a curare-like anticholinesterase effect and by competing with calcium; this is more likely to be seen following the use of muscle relaxants during anaesthesia.

Kidneys

Since the kidneys are the major route of drug excretion, it is not surprising that nephrotoxicity is relatively frequent. It is often dose related and is more common either in those with pre-existing renal failure or in those receiving other nephrotoxic agents.

Sulphonamides

Some early sulphonamides, which were rapidly excreted and poorly soluble, were prone to deposit crystals within the urinary tract, sometimes causing tubular damage and ureteric obstruction. This is uncommon with later sulphonamides, which are generally more soluble and more slowly excreted. A similar complication has been linked to the protease inhibitors indinavir and ritonavir, used in the treatment of HIV infection.

Tetracyclines

These may occasionally be nephrotoxic, particularly in patients with pre-existing renal insufficiency and older people with physiological renal impairment. The degree of renal failure varies, but is usually reversible. An explanation of the phenomenon may lie in the anti-anabolic effect of tetracyclines.

A specific effect of demeclocycline is the production of nephrogenic diabetes insipidus, a phenomenon that has been put to therapeutic advantage in the management of the syndrome of inappropriate antidiuretic hormone secretion.

Among tetracyclines, doxycycline is unique in being devoid of nephrotoxicity, reflecting its primary hepatobiliary route of excretion.

Aminoglycosides

These are the antibiotics most frequently associated with nephrotoxicity. Their nephrotoxic potential varies and occurs in decreasing order of frequency with gentamicin, tobramycin, amikacin, and netilmicin. Nephrotoxicity is potentiated by pre-existing renal disease, prolonged or repeated courses of treatment, or the simultaneous administration of other nephrotoxic agents. Renal damage is often reversible, although permanent impairment including renal failure does occur.

Amphotericin B

Nephrotoxicity is the leading complication of the use of amphotericin B. This results from a combination of a reduction in glomerular filtration, renal tubular acidosis, and decreased concentrating ability. Careful monitoring of renal function is a prerequisite to the use of this agent. Lipid formulations of amphotericin B (p. 70) are less nephrotoxic.

Haematological toxicity

Bone marrow toxicity may be selective and affect one cell line, or be unselective and produce pancytopenia and marrow aplasia. Immune-mediated haemolysis, in which Coombs' antibodies are detected, may also occur. Bleeding may occur from platelet dysfunction or from thrombo-cytopenia. Eosinophilia may represent a hypersensitivity reaction.

β-Lactam antibiotics

The penicillins may rarely produce a primary haemolytic anaemia and Coombs' antibody-positive disease. Selective white cell depression has been described with ampicillin and flucloxacillin. Similarly, the cephalospor-ins may be associated with a positive Coombs' test, although frank haemolysis is uncommon. Eosinophilia occurs with variable frequency, as does the selective depression of white cells, and occasionally platelets, following the development of platelet antibodies. A vitamin K-dependent bleeding disorder has been associated with cephalosporins possessing a thiotetrazole side-chain, such as cefamandole, cefotetan, and cefoperazone. Although uncommon, bleeding occurs in elderly or malnourished patients undergoing major surgery. It is both treated and prevented by the administration of vitamin K.

Sulphonamides

Among the more important groups of agents to produce haematological side effects are the sulphonamides and sulphonamide-containing mixtures such as co-trimoxazole. Marrow toxicity may result in aplastic anaemia, or a selective neutropenia, or thrombocytopenia. In addition, haemolysis may be either primary or related to glucose-6-phosphate dehydrogenase deficiency. Co-trimoxazole may produce megaloblastic bone marrow changes or, less commonly, a peripheral megaloblastic anaemia. This tends to occur with prolonged therapy and is related to the joint antifolate action of the two components of co-trimoxazole.

Chloramphenicol

This has achieved notoriety for inducing marrow depression, which is manifested in two ways. The more common dose-related bone marrow depression is seen when the daily dose exceeds 4 g. There is a progressive anaemia, neutropenia, and sometimes thrombocytopenia, which is reversible on either discontinuing treatment or reducing the dosage. A more serious reaction is that of total bone marrow depression and aplastic anaemia. This is unpredictable but is estimated to occur with a frequency of 1 in 24 000 to 1 in 40 000 treatment courses. Mortality from aplastic anaemia is in excess of 50%. Thiamphenicol, a derivative of chloramphenicol available in some parts of the world, appears to be devoid of the irreversible toxic effects on the bone marrow.

Adverse reactions to antiviral drugs

The past decade has seen the licensing of many new antiviral drugs, largely for the treatment of herpesviruses and HIV infections. Inevitably this has led to the recognition of a range of adverse reactions, some of which are unique to this class of agents.

Antiherpesvirus agents

Aciclovir has proved remarkably free from serious toxicity. However, if administered in high dosage crystal deposition in the renal tubules can occur, occasionally leading to renal failure, unless patients are kept adequately hydrated. Neurotoxicity manifested by tremor, ataxia, and seizures can also complicate high dosage treatment or administration to patients with renal impairment. These side effects usually resolve on stopping treatment.

Ganciclovir, in contrast to aciclovir, is a more toxic drug. The major complication of use is bone marrow suppression, particularly neutropenia. This can prove difficult to manage since the drug is often required to treat cytomegalovirus infection in bone marrow and organ transplanted patients. Such patients are already extremely immunosuppressed and any additional drug-induced bone marrow suppression is undesirable. Foscarnet is an alternative to ganciclovir for the treatment of cytomegalovirus infections. While it is not associated with bone marrow suppression, its major adverse effect is dose related renal impairment. This requires careful monitoring of renal function during treatment, with dose reduction and sometimes cessation of therapy. An unusual complication is genital ulceration.

Antiretroviral agents

This group of agents has expanded rapidly over the past 15 years. The clinical trials programme has often been accelerated resulting in early licensing before the full range of adverse reactions has been defined. Furthermore, the potential for interaction both between these agents and between other classes of drugs, is high and they therefore require considerable caution and expertise in their use. A selection of side effects to commonly used agents is provided.

Nucleoside reverse transcriptase inhibitors

Zidovudine (AZT) was the first antiretroviral drug to be approved and is still in widespread use. Bone marrow suppression primarily causing mild to moderate anaemia is the most common side effect. This tends to be macrocytic in nature since the drug is less suppressive to early immature forms of erythrocytes, than the mature red cell. Other side effects include myopathy, hepatotoxicity, and pigmentation of the nails.

Didanosine and stavudine can both cause a sensory neuropathy, often starting in the feet. Unless detected early, it can progress to produce severe paraesthesiae and sensory loss. Another unusual yet serious adverse effect of these drugs is acute pancreatitis. Careful monitoring and measurement of serum amylase can avoid this complication. Bone marrow toxicity may also occur.

Abacavir is a potent drug but may cause a severe hypersensitivity reaction, which precludes continued use. Skin rashes can also be troublesome.

Lamivudine is widely prescribed and generally safe. Pancreatitis occurs rarely.

Non-nucleoside reverse transcriptase inhibitors

Nevirapine is most commonly linked to early onset skin rashes. These occur in approximately 20% of patients within the first month of treatment and in a small number are severe and life threatening especially causing the Stevens–Johnson syndrome. Nevirapine is a potent inducer of the cytochrome P-450 enzymes; drugs such as rifampicin and rifabutin require dose adjustment if co-administered.

Efavirenz frequently causes mild to moderate neuropsychiatric side effects in the first few weeks of treatment. These include anxiety, insomnia, vivid dreams, depression and, rarely, a suicidal response.

Protease inhibitors

Saquinavir is generally well tolerated but notorious for interactions with other agents. It increases the plasma concentrations of terfenamide and astemizole, while other drugs either reduce plasma concentrations of saquinavir (rifampicin, rifabutin) or increase them (ketoconazole, ritonavir). The interaction with ritonavir has been exploited pharmaceutically, since it is often co-marketed in fixed dose formulations of other protease inhibitors (e.g. lopinavir + ritonavir) to boost their plasma concentrations to therapeutic advantage.

Nelfinavir is associated with dose-related mild to moderate diarrhoea.

Prevention of adverse reactions

There are major difficulties in preventing adverse drug reactions. Patients frequently respond idiosyncratically to antimicrobial agents, as to other drugs; the chief problem, especially with the rarer side effects, is their unpredictability. Awareness of the possibility of adverse effects is obviously important, and a close working relationship with either a clinical pharmacist or a specialist in the use of antimicrobial agents will help to overcome problems as they arise.

When toxic effects develop or are suspected, the decision has to be made whether to stop or change the patient's treatment. The drug may often be continued provided the dose is adjusted by reducing each individual dose or by prolonging the interval between doses.

Antibiotic assays are important in determining whether dosage adjustment is necessary, particularly in the case of aminoglycosides, in which the leeway between effective and toxic levels is small.

Finally, the reporting of adverse drug reactions, whether caused by antimicrobial agents or other drugs, remains the responsibility of all practising doctors. In the UK the Medicines and Healthcare Products Regulatory Agency's Committee on Safety of Medicines operates a voluntary adverse reactions reporting system (see Postscript, p. 452).

Chapter 17

Chemoprophylaxis

Chemoprophylaxis is the prevention of infection by the administration of antimicrobial agents as distinct from prevention by immunization. Individuals who require prophylaxis differ from the normal population in that they are known to be exposed to a particular infectious hazard or their ability to respond to infection is impaired.

Prophylaxis should be confined to those periods for which the risk is greatest, so that the problems of disturbance of the normal flora, superinfection with resistant organisms, untoward reactions, and cost will be minimized. The benefits and risks of chemoprophylaxis depend on:

- the likelihood of infection in the absence of prophylaxis;
- the potential severity of the consequences of infection;
- the effectiveness of prophylaxis in reducing the likelihood of infection and the severity of the consequences;
- the likelihood and consequences of adverse effects from prophylaxis.

Prevention strategies for infectious disease can be characterized by the traditional concepts of primary, secondary, and tertiary prevention. *Primary prevention* can be defined as the prevention of infection. *Secondary prevention* includes measures for the detection of early infection and effective intervention before symptoms occur. *Tertiary prevention* consists of measures to reduce or eliminate the long-term impairment and disabilities caused by established infection.

Failure to consider fully the risks of prophylaxis or to be realistic about the benefits has made unnecessary chemoprophylaxis one of the commonest forms of antibiotic misuse. None the less it is important to recognize that the judgement about what is and is not necessary chemoprophylaxis may require complex decisions about the balance of benefits and risks to individual patients and to the population. The example of prevention of neonatal infection by Group B Streptococci (see below) shows how national guidelines committees can produce different recommendations based on their risk assessment of the same evidence.

Primary chemoprophylaxis

Most indications for primary chemoprophylaxis involve starting prophylaxis before a period of defined risk (e.g. elective surgery or travel to regions with endemic malaria or intrapartum exposure of neonates to maternal infections) or following exposure to a patient who is known to have a contagious, dangerous infection (e.g. meningococcal meningitis).

Prophylaxis in surgery

Reducing the risk of surgical infection is probably the commonest indication for chemoprophylaxis and accounts for up to a third of total antibiotic use in an acute hospital. There is no doubt that prophylaxis can reduce the risk of surgical infection but at best it is only one component of effective infection control and unnecessary use of prophylaxis puts patients at risk of infection by *Clostridium difficile* or antimicrobial resistant bacteria with no compensating benefit.

Classification of operations by risk of infection

The aim of chemoprophylaxis is to reduce the risk of surgical site infection, meaning infection in any part of the operative field from the superficial wound down to the deepest tissues involved in the operation. Postoperative infections can occur at other sites, for example the respiratory or urinary tract but chemoprophylaxis is targeted at surgical site infection.

The probability of surgical site infection is determined by the risk of contamination of the wound, the patient's general health, and the duration of the operation. Risk of contamination is defined by classifying wounds as clean, clean contaminated, contaminated, or dirty (Table 17.1). Primary prevention by chemoprophylaxis is only achievable for clean, clean-contaminated, or contaminated wounds because the process of infection has started pre-operatively in dirty wounds. The risk of infection rises progressively with the degree of contamination of the wound; however, the patient's co-morbidities and duration of surgery are equally important determinants (Table 17.2). A prolonged operation with a clean wound in a patient with co-morbidities carries a 5% risk of wound infection, substantially higher than the 3.5% risk for a contaminated wound in a patient with no co-morbidities and a short operation (Table 17.2).

In addition to the probability that an infection will occur it is important to consider the consequences of infection for the patient and the health service. Surgical site infection following colon surgery is associated with substantially increased risk of mortality and prophylaxis significantly reduces death within

Prevention of Antimicrobial Resistance: guidelines for the prevention of antimicrobial resistance in hospitals. *Clinical Infectious Diseases* 1997; **25**: 584–599.

Woodford EM, Wilson KA, Marriott JF. Documentation of antimicrobial prescribing controls in UK NHS hospitals. *Journal of Antimicrobial Chemotherapy* 2004; **53**: 650–652.

Part 4

Therapeutic use of antimicrobial agents

Chapter 19

Respiratory tract infections

Respiratory infections are caused by viruses, or bacteria, or both. If the illness is entirely viral in origin, an antibiotic will not help. If there is a bacterial component, antibiotic treatment will sometimes help, and may be vital. It is often difficult to recognize when bacteria may be involved in respiratory infection as secondary bacterial infection may complicate viral respiratory infections. However, the key question in the decision about treatment with antimicrobials is: do the benefits to the patient outweigh the risks? It is not necessary to prescribe antimicrobials for all bacterial respiratory infections.

When considering the role of antimicrobial chemotherapy it is important to reflect on the epidemiology of infection in the twentieth century (Fig. 19.1). There are two striking features: the doubling of mortality in 1918, caused by the influenza pandemic; and the steep decline in mortality through the first half of the century, before the arrival of antimicrobial chemotherapy or vaccines. The introduction of antimicrobial chemotherapy did accelerate the decline in mortality from some respiratory infections

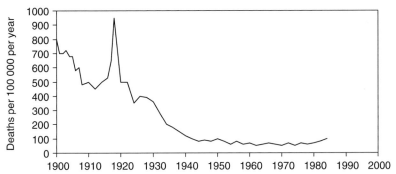

Fig. 19.1 Infectious diseases mortality in the USA during the twentieth century. Reproduced from Armstrong GL, Conn LA, Pinner RW. Trends in infectious disease mortality in the United States during the 20th century. *Journal of the American Medical Association* 1999; **28**: 61–66 with permission from American Medical Association.

(e.g. otitis media, pneumonia, and tuberculosis) but had no impact on others (e.g. bronchitis). Two conclusions can be drawn from Fig. 19.1 first, it is clear why there is so much concern about the possibility of an influenza pandemic given the massive impact on mortality of the 1918 pandemic. Second, antimicrobial chemotherapy has not had the dramatic effect on mortality from infections that is popularly attributed to it. The major impact in the first half of the twentieth century came from improvements in public health, which is why death from all infections still increases with increasing socio-economic deprivation in the twenty-first century. Antimicrobial chemotherapy is just one component of an overall strategy to prevent and treat infections.

Upper respiratory tract infection

Sore throat

This is one of the commonest acute problems seen in general medical practice, with an incidence of 100 cases per 1000 inhabitants per year, although only a minority of these will present to a doctor. It is commoner in females than men. Symptoms include: sore throat with anorexia, lethargy, and systemic illness. On examination there may be inflamed tonsils or pharynx, a purulent exudate on tonsils, fever, and anterior cervical lymphadenopathy.

Sore throat may be part of the early symptom complex of many upper respiratory viral infections, in which case cough is a common additional feature. Occasionally, it may be a presenting symptom of acute epiglottitis or other serious upper airway disease.

There is no evidence that bacterial sore throats are more severe or long-lasting than viral ones. The most commonly identified organism is *Streptococcus pyogenes*, the group A β-haemolytic streptococcus. Most other cases are caused by adenoviruses. There is no reliable way to distinguish between bacterial and viral causes based on symptoms and signs.

The gold standard for diagnosis of streptococcal infection in the throat includes a positive anti-streptolysin O (ASO) titre in addition to culture of *Str. pyogenes* from the throat. There is a high asymptomatic carrier rate for the organism (up to 40%) and it is common to culture it from sore throats when there is no serological evidence of infection. Moreover a negative culture does not rule out *Str. pyogenes* as a cause of sore throat. Neither culture of throat swabs nor rapid tests based on detection of streptococcal antigen are helpful in most cases.

Most people with sore throat manage the condition successfully without seeing a doctor. Paracetamol is an effective analgesic, with less risk of adverse effects than non-steroidal anti-inflammatory drugs. Aspirin should be avoided in children because of the risk of Reye's syndrome. The immediate benefits from antimicrobial chemotherapy are actually very meagre. Symptoms usually persist for 5–7 days with or without antibiotics, which only shorten illness by 24 h. The same control of symptoms can probably be achieved with paracetamol.

Streptococcal sore throat is important because it may lead to serious complications, particularly rheumatic fever, which is still prevalent in many countries. Evidence about the effectiveness of antibiotics for preventing non-suppurative and suppurative complications comes from studies on military personnel living in overcrowded barracks in the late 1940s and early 1950s. This evidence has little relevance to management of sore throat in modern communities, at least in the developed world, where rheumatic fever is now very uncommon. Similarly experience with the use of antibiotics to prevent cross-infection in sore throat comes mainly from army barracks and other closed institutions. It is very unlikely (and unproven) that trying to eradicate *Str. pyogenes* with routine antibiotic therapy for sore throat will produce any measurable health gain in the general public in Western countries, whereas it is likely that this would increase the prevalence of antimicrobial resistance.

A patient information leaflet may be of value in the management of acute sore throat and may assist in managing future episodes at home without general practitioner involvement. Patients who are sceptical about with-holding antibiotics can be given a prescription with the suggestion that they do not use it unless their symptoms persist for more than 3 days. Only about 30% of patients who are given delayed prescriptions go to the pharmacy to get their antibiotics.

If antibiotics are to be prescribed the drugs of choice are penicillin V or a macrolide, and these should be given for at least 10 days to eradicate the organism and prevent recurrence. Glandular fever commonly causes symptoms and signs that are indistinguishable from streptococcal throat infection (including a very impressive purulent exudate on the tonsils). Ampicillin, amoxicillin, and co-amoxiclav should not be used, as they will cause a rash if the sore throat is the herald of glandular fever. Tetracyclines are also inappropriate because of the high incidence of resistance among streptococci.

Other infections that may present with sore throat

Croup

Noisy difficult breathing, hoarseness, and stridor are common signs of croup, a distressing condition that is usually viral in origin. Treatment is supportive; the condition is usually self-limiting and resolves in 2–4 days if uncomplicated, but severe cases may require endotracheal intubation or tracheostomy. Acute epiglottitis is a much less common, but much more dangerous, cause of croup caused by infection with *Haemophilus influenzae* type b; it can occur in adults as well as in children. There is systemic illness as well as local respiratory difficulty, and the swollen oedematous epiglottis can cause complete airways obstruction with dramatic suddenness. It is this complication that makes acute epiglottitis such a life-threatening condition. Treatment is as much concerned with maintaining the airways as with controlling the infection.

If breathing difficulty is present in a patient with croup, urgent referral to hospital is mandatory and attempts to examine the throat should be avoided.

Diphtheria

Although rare in countries with effective vaccination policies, diphtheria is still prevalent in many parts of the world. Diagnosis is made on clinical grounds, notably the presence of a characteristic membranous exudate on the tonsils and pharynx. Treatment with antitoxin should be given immediately without waiting for laboratory confirmation. Antibiotics have no part to play in treating the infection, but penicillin or erythromycin is effective in eradicating the infection to prevent spread.

Thrush

Oral thrush, infection of the mucous membrane with the yeast *Candida albicans*, is predominantly a neonatal infection. Candida is a common vaginal commensal, especially in pregnancy, and the infant acquires infection during passage through the birth canal. It presents in the first few days of life as white curdy patches on cheeks, lips, palate, and tongue. Treatment is with local nystatin.

In adults, oral thrush may follow treatment with antibacterials or corticosteroids. However, it may be indicative of serious underlying disease, such as diabetes or immunodeficiency (Chapter 28). In all these conditions one of the oral polyene or azole derivatives may be used to control the candida.

Acute otitis media

Three-quarters of cases of acute otitis media occur in children; one in four children will have an episode during their first 10 years of life. Acute otitis media should be distinguished from otitis media with effusion, commonly referred to as glue ear; as many as 80% of children suffer this infection at least once before the age of 4.

Acute otitis media is an inflammation of the middle ear of rapid onset presenting with local symptoms (earache, rubbing or tugging of the affected ear) and systemic signs (fever, irritability, disturbed sleeping). It is often preceded by other upper respiratory symptoms such as cough or rhinorrhoea. On examination a middle ear effusion may be present but in addition the drum looks opaque and may be bulging.

The condition is caused predominantly by *H. influenzae* and *Streptococcus pneumoniae*. Staphylococci, *Str. pyogenes*, and α-haemolytic streptococci are less often involved. However, acute otitis media should not be treated routinely with antibiotics. As with sore throat, antibiotics only have a small impact on the duration of acute symptoms, which can be controlled equally effective with paracetamol. If an antibiotic is to be prescribed a 5-day course is sufficient; the antibiotic of choice is amoxicillin; erythromycin and co-amoxiclav are logical alternatives and may be necessary if β-lactamase-producing *H. influenzae* is involved. Decongestants, antihistamines, and mucolytics are not effective. As with sore throat, patient information leaflets and delayed antibiotic prescriptions are effective strategies for reducing the unnecessary use of antibiotics.

Glue ear is an inflammation of the middle ear with accumulation of fluid in the middle ear but without symptoms or signs of acute inflammation. It is often asymptomatic and earache is uncommon. On examination a middle ear effusion is present but with a normal looking ear drum. Antibiotics should not be given.

Acute sinusitis

Acute sinusitis presents with pain originating in the maxillary, frontal, ethmoid, or sphenoid sinuses, with the maxillary sinus being by far the commonest. Onset of facial pain is often preceded by non-specific symptoms of upper respiratory inflammation and there may be systemic signs of inflammation. The bacterial causes of acute sinusitis are the same as acute otitis media. If X-ray or culture confirms the clinical diagnosis then antibiotics can substantially reduce the duration of symptoms. However, neither of these investigations is routinely available in primary care.

Culture of the sinuses requires percutaneous sinus puncture and aspiration, which is not a procedure that most general practitioners are trained to do (or that many patients would consent to). Unfortunately antibiotic treatment of patients with symptoms suggestive of sinusitis but without confirmation by X-ray or culture is no more effective than symptomatic relief.

As with acute otitis media antibiotics for acute sinusitis should be reserved for the more severe cases. Penicillin V or amoxicillin are as effective as newer antibiotics. The recommended duration of treatment is 10 days in the absence of evidence that shorter courses are as effective.

Lower respiratory tract infections

Acute cough is the most common symptom of lower respiratory infection, whether as a new symptom or as an exacerbation of chronic symptoms. Cough is not a universal feature: some patients with pneumonia present with pleuritic chest pain or with symptoms of systemic inflammatory response (fever, malaise, headache, or myalgia) without cough. The most important diagnosis to make is pneumonia because it can be life threatening and its outcome can be improved with antimicrobial chemotherapy. However, it is not possible to distinguish reliably between pneumonia and other causes of lower respiratory tract infection from clinical history and signs. Consequently, in primary care management must be based on an assessment of severity of illness and need for referral to hospital.

Epidemiology

The incidence of lower respiratory tract infection in the UK is between 40 and 90 cases per 1000 population per year, being commoner in the very young and old and in the winter months. In the UK there is about a fourfold higher incidence in the most deprived communities in comparison with the most affluent communities.

Mortality is highest in the elderly. The 30-day mortality associated with lower respiratory tract infection in people over 65 years old is 10%. However, many of these elderly people die 'with' rather than 'of' the infection. Bronchopneumonia is often recorded as the immediate cause of death in people with chronic, life-threatening diseases. Mortality from 'pneumonia' has actually increased in developed countries since the introduction of antibiotics, but more people are living longer and most of this mortality is from bronchopneumonia.

Most people with lower respiratory infections manage their own symptoms without seeking medical attention. Of 1 million people with lower respiratory tract infection only 300 000 will see a primary care physician. Of these 1 in 4 (70 000) will be treated with antibiotics, although only about 1 in 10 (7000 people) will have a diagnosis of pneumonia. From the original 300 000 people who presented to a primary care physician only about 200 (0.7%) will be admitted to hospital with pneumonia.

Management in primary care

The key to management of lower respiratory tract infection in primary care is to distinguish between patients who have severe infection that should be referred to hospital and the majority (99%) who can be managed safely at home. There are four questions to address:

- Has the patient been previously well or is there underlying chronic respiratory or other disease?
- Has there been the development or deterioration in either dyspnoea or sputum purulence?
- Are there any new localizing physical signs in the chest to suggest pneumonia?
- Are any features of severity present (Box 19.1).

The answers to these questions distinguish between four broad populations of people with lower respiratory tract infection. These will be discussed starting with the most severe (but least common).

Box 19.1 Features of severity of lower respiratory tract infection that can be easily assessed in primary care (items in bold are most important)

- **Raised respiratory rate (>30/min)**
- **Low blood pressure (<90 mmHg systolic and or <60 mmHg diastolic)**
- **Confusion of recent onset**
- **Age >50 years**
- Coexisting disease present (e.g. severe chronic obstructive pulmonary disease, cardiac failure, cerebrovascular, neoplastic, renal or liver disease)
- Very high or very low temperature ($<35°C$ or $>40°C$)
- Tachycardia (>125/min)

Patients with features indicating severe infection

Referral to hospital should be considered in patients who exhibit one or more of the features of severity (Box 19.1), especially if they are over the age of 50. This applies whether or not the patient has additional physical signs indicating pneumonia because the absence of these signs is not a reliable method for excluding pneumonia. The final decision should be based on clinical judgement that includes social factors. Even a relatively well patient who lives in poor social circumstances or in an isolated rural area with no home support may require referral to hospital. Conversely patients who are 65 years old and have signs of pneumonia can be managed safely at home if they have sufficient social support.

Suspected community-acquired pneumonia without features of severity

These patients have new focal signs in the chest (crackles or altered breath sounds), but are not severely ill. In the absence of chest X-ray (not available in many primary care settings) pneumonia can be diagnosed from symptoms of an acute lower respiratory infection (cough or dyspnoea or pleuritic chest pain) with at least one systemic symptom of infection (fever or tachycardia) and new focal signs on chest examination. However, only 50% of those with all of these features will actually have an abnormal chest X-ray.

Below the age of 45 very few patients with pneumonia also have chronic obstructive pulmonary disease. Between the ages of 45 and 64 the proportion is up to 10% and rises to 20% between the ages of 75 and 84. Pneumonia in these patients is more likely to be associated with severity criteria (Box 19.1).

A wide variety of organisms can cause pneumonia, including viruses. The commonest bacterial cause is *Str. pneumoniae*, which accounts for about 70–80% of cases in which a bacterial pathogen is identified. Atypical bacteria (*Mycoplasma pneumoniae*, *Chlamydophila* (*Chlamydia*) *pneumoniae*, *Chlamydophila psittaci*, *Legionella pneumophila*, and *Coxiella burnetii*) collectively account for 10–20% of cases and the remainder are caused by *H. influenzae* or *Staphylococcus aureus*. The latter is particularly associated with secondary bacterial infection following influenza.

With current technology neither sputum culture nor blood tests such as C-reactive protein or white cell count provide sufficient added value to the diagnosis to justify routine use. Sputum culture may be recommended in areas with a high prevalence of penicillin-resistant pneumococci.

Pneumonia is a life-threatening illness. None the less, patients with no features of severity (Box 19.1) can be managed safely at home with oral amoxicillin, a macrolide, or a tetracycline. There is no need to give combination therapy. A macrolide or tetracycline may be preferred if there are clinical features suggesting infection with one of the atypical bacteria (e.g. prominent upper respiratory symptoms, headache, or symptom duration for >1 week) particularly in younger patients or during an epidemic year for *M. pneumoniae*.

Patients with underlying chronic respiratory disease

These patients often have no new signs in the chest other than dyspnoea and sputum purulence. In the absence of signs of severity (Box 19.1) or of pneumonia the diagnosis is an acute exacerbation of the underlying condition. The likely bacterial pathogens are *H. influenzae*, *Str. pneumoniae*, and *Moraxella catarrhalis*. The development of green (purulent) sputum is a good indicator of a high bacterial load in the sputum. However, even in these patients antibacterial treatment has only a slight impact on the course of an acute exacerbation, shortening an illness of 5–7 days by no more than 1 day. Antibacterial treatment does not benefit patients with acute exacerbations of chronic obstructive pulmonary disease who do not have purulent sputum. The prevalence of resistance to aminopenicillins in *H. influenzae* is 10–30% and is much higher in *Mor. catarrhalis*. Despite this the clinical effectiveness of amoxicillin is just as good as co-amoxiclav or fluoroquinolones, probably because of the modest benefit from any antibacterial treatment. For the same reason routine sputum culture is not recommended and should be reserved for patients with symptoms that persist despite treatment with amoxicillin. A macrolide or tetracycline is appropriate for patients who are allergic to penicillin, or who have not responded to amoxicillin treatment. Fluoroquinolones should not be used empirically in the management of exacerbations of respiratory disease in primary care.

Non-pneumonic lower respiratory infection (acute bronchitis)

Most patients with no signs in the chest, who have been previously well and do not have other features of severity, have non-pneumonic infection, most of which are caused by viruses. A few cases are caused by *M. pneumoniae*, *Bordetella pertussis*, *C. pneumoniae*, *Str. pneumoniae*, or *H. influenzae*. Patients will have an illness lasting several days with or without antibiotics, which should not be prescribed unless patients have signs in the chest or features of severity (Box 19.1). Sputum purulence alone is not an indication for antibiotics in a previously well patient with no chest signs. As with sore throat and acute otitis media, patient information leaflets and delayed prescriptions are effective strategies for reducing unnecessary antibiotic treatment.

Pertussis (whooping cough)

Antibiotics are notoriously ineffective in controlling the distressing cough of pertussis; nevertheless, erythromycin has been shown to eradicate the organism from the respiratory tract and can also be used for the protection of susceptible close contacts. Vaccination is the only reliable way of preventing and controlling this early childhood infectious disease.

Cystic fibrosis

The susceptibility of patients with cystic fibrosis to pulmonary infection is well recognized and is often the cause of early death. Most lung infections in patients with cystic fibrosis are managed in the community, usually by outreach teams from secondary care. One of the striking features of chest infections in cystic fibrosis is that relatively few pathogens are involved. Early in the disease the organisms implicated are frequently *Staph. aureus* or *H. influenzae*, or both. As patients progress through adolescence to adulthood, these pathogens are replaced by *Pseudomonas aeruginosa*. Major problems arise when *Ps. aeruginosa* is replaced by *Stenotrophomonas maltophilia* or *Burkholderia cepacia*; these organisms are often resistant to many antibiotics and treatment should be guided by laboratory findings. The selection of antibiotics in patients with cystic fibrosis should be determined by the specialist services that manage the patient.

Management in hospital

Community-acquired pneumonia

In hospital the clinical diagnosis can be confirmed with a chest X-ray, although it should be recognized that its sensitivity is not 100%. The gold standard for diagnosis of bacterial pneumonia is culture of bacteria from lung tissues or a needle aspirate from the lung but these tests are too dangerous to use in routine clinical practice. The point is that some patients with pneumonia can have a normal chest X-ray at presentation, so if the clinical features strongly suggest pneumonia it is reasonable to treat and repeat the chest X-ray after 24–48 h.

The severity criteria for community-acquired pneumonia are based on assessments of confusion, urea concentration, respiratory rate, and blood pressure for those 65 years of age and older (CURB-65 score; Table 19.1). It is similar to but importantly different from the classification of severity of sepsis (Chapter 13, p. 185). The CURB-65 score is specifically designed to

Table 19.1 The CURB-65 severity score for patients presenting to hospital with community acquired pneumonia and the mortality range measured in two prospective cohort studies. CURB-65: score one point for each of: Confusion; urea >7 mmol/l; respiratory rate ≥30/min; low systolic (<90 mm Hg) or diastolic (≤60 mm Hg) blood pressure); age ≥65 years

Risk	CURB-65 score	30-day mortality
Low risk	0–1	0–1%
Intermediate	2	8–9%
High risk	>2	22–23%
All patients	Not applicable	9–10%

Data from Lim WS, van der Eerden MM, Laing R, Boersma WG, Karalus N, Town GI, Lewis SA, Macfarlane JT. Defining community acquired pneumonia severity on presentation to hospital: an international derivation and validation study. *Thorax* 2003; **58**: 377–382.

be used in patients who present to hospital in order to identify low-risk patients who do not need to be admitted to hospital, whereas the classification of sepsis is intended to be used for any patient with infection (community or hospital acquired) to identify patients who are deteriorating and require more intensive therapy. The CURB-65 score identifies low-risk patients more accurately than the sepsis severity score. There are more complex pneumonia-specific scores (for example the pneumonia severity index used in North America) but these are no more accurate than CURB-65.

Between 30 and 50% of patients who present to hospital with community-acquired pneumonia are found to be in the CURB-65 low-risk group. However, about half of these patients have other reasons for admission. Some will have co-morbidities that require inpatient management. In particular, patients with chronic obstructive pulmonary disease and pneumonia could be in respiratory failure and yet have a CURB-65 score of 0 (if they have a respiratory rate <30/min, which is likely if they have Type 2 respiratory failure). In addition to medical reasons for admission some patients will have poor social circumstances or insufficient support to be managed at home.

The management of patients admitted to hospital should be determined by their CURB-65 score. Low-risk patients who are admitted for other reasons can be managed in the same way as low-risk patients in the community, with either amoxicillin, a macrolide, or a tetracycline. Some guidelines do recommend that all patients admitted to hospital with pneumonia should receive antibiotics for pneumonia caused by atypical bacteria but several clinical trials shows that treatment with an aminopenicillin alone is just as effective for patients with low or intermediate risk pneumonia.

At the other end of the scale, patients at high risk should be treated with intravenous antibiotics that are effective against the full range of pathogens that may cause community-acquired pneumonia. Possible regimens include co-amoxiclav or cefuroxime plus a macrolide, or a fluoroquinolone with good activity against *Str. pneumoniae* (e.g. levofloxacin). The patient must receive the antibiotic(s) immediately and certainly within 4 h of admission as later administration is associated with increased mortality. If patients are admitted through an Accident and Emergency Department they must receive their first dose of antibiotics there before transfer to the ward. If they are admitted direct to a ward the first dose must be clearly written for immediate administration, not left until the next drug round. In addition to intravenous antibiotics patients with severe pneumonia must have their oxygen require-ments assessed by pulse oximetry or blood gas measurement within 4 h of admission and receive high flow oxygen (5 litres per minute) if they are hypoxic. Adequate fluid replacement is also essential. Patients should be referred to a high dependency or intensive care unit if their vital signs do not improve rapidly. When young patients die from community-acquired pneumonia it is usually because of failure to recognize the need for intensive care.

The management of patients at intermediate risk falls between these two extremes and is a matter for clinical judgement. If in doubt it would be wise to treat as severe pneumonia while waiting for senior review.

Hospital-acquired pneumonia

Pneumonia is the leading cause of mortality resulting from infection acquired in hospital. The incidence of hospital-acquired pneumonia in intensive care units ranges from 10 to 65%, with case fatalities of 13–55%. It is often associated with mechanical ventilation. The risk of hospital-acquired pneumonia can be substantially reduced by using non-invasive methods for respiratory support instead of ventilation and by having clear care protocols for protecting host defences against respiratory infection during mechanical ventilation. Chemoprophylaxis plays a role through the use of selective decontamination of the digestive tract (see p. 241), which reduces the numbers of Gram-negative bacilli and hence the risk of infection.

The micro-organisms causing pneumonia within 5 days of admission are quite different from those seen in disease with a later onset. The bacteria responsible for early onset pneumonia are *Str. pneumoniae, H. influenzae, Staph. aureus,* and only rarely enteric Gram-negative bacilli. In contrast late onset infection is almost always caused by Gram-negative bacteria, mainly enterobacteria but also *Ps. aeruginosa* and *Acinetobacter spp.*

Methicillin-resistant *Staph. aureus* (MRSA) is becoming increasingly common in some units. Since tracheal aspirates are poor indicators of the cause of ventilator-associated pneumonia, bronchoalveolar lavage is recommended to confirm the diagnosis.

Empirical treatment for early onset pneumonia in patients who have not received antibiotics should be with co-amoxiclav or cefuroxime. Treatment of patients who have already received antibiotics or have late onset disease should be with a broad-spectrum cephalosporin such as cefotaxime, a fluoroquinolone or piperacillin plus tazobactam. Combination therapy is no more effective than monotherapy. Subsequent treatment should be directed by the results of broncho-alveolar lavage.

Other respiratory tract infections

Pneumonia developing in association with neutropenia following treatment with cytotoxic drugs, or in patients with immunosuppression, including those suffering from AIDS, may be due to *Pneumocystis carinii*, other fungi, or viruses. Appropriate treatment is discussed in Chapters 27 and 28. The treatment of tuberculosis is considered in Chapter 25; influenza and other respiratory viral infections are dealt with in Chapter 27.

Further reading

British Society for Antimicrobial Chemotherapy guidelines for hospital acquired pneumonia, *Journal of Antimicrobial Chemotherapy* in press 2006.

British Thoracic Society. British Thoracic Society guidelines for the management of community acquired pneumonia in childhood. *Thorax* 2002; **57** Suppl 1: i1–i24. Available at: http://thorax.bmjjournals.com/cgi/content/full/57/90001/i1

British Thoracic Society. British Thoracic Society guidelines for the management of community acquired pneumonia in adults. *Thorax* 2001; **56** Suppl 4: iv1–iv64. Available at: http://thorax.bmjjournals.com/cgi/content/full/56/suppl_4/iv1

British Thoracic Society. British Thoracic Society guidelines for the management of community acquired pneumonia in adults–2004 Update. Available at: http://www.brit-thoracic.org.uk/c2/uploads/MACAPrevisedApr04.pdf

Metlay JP, Fine MJ. Testing strategies in the initial management of patients with community-acquired pneumonia. *Annals of Internal Medicine* 2003; **138**: 109–118.

Scottish Intercollegiate Guidelines Network (www.sign.ac.uk)

Guideline 34: management of sore throat and indications for tonsillectomy

Guideline 66: diagnosis and management of childhood otitis media in primary care

Guideline 59: community management of lower respiratory tract infection in adults

Antibiotic treatment

Symptomatic infection

Patients with symptomatic infection of the lower or upper urinary tract benefit from antibiotic treatment. Symptoms would resolve without antibiotic treatment in about 50% of people with lower urinary tract infection but they resolve much faster with antibiotic treatment. Patients with symptoms of upper urinary tract infection require urgent effective antibiotic treatment to minimize the risk of bacteraemia.

In general practice about half the women presenting with frequency and dysuria have sterile urine cultures. This condition is sometimes referred to as the 'urethral syndrome' or symptomatic abacteriuria—a common, but largely unexplained condition. Some cases may be due to sexually transmitted organisms, such as chlamydia, and some may represent the early stages of urinary infection. Counselling is more important than antimicrobial therapy, but persistent symptoms need further investigation.

Asymptomatic bacteriuria

There are only two groups of patients in whom asymptomatic bacteriuria should be treated with antibiotics:

1. In very young children whose kidneys are still growing there is evidence that asymptomatic bacteriuria is associated with scarring of the kidney and predisposes to hypertension or chronic renal impairment. Young children who have had symptomatic urinary tract infection are therefore followed up after treatment to ensure that they do not have continuing bacteriuria.

2. In pregnancy asymptomatic bacteriuria is associated with increased risk of pyelonephritis later in pregnancy and with pre-term delivery. Moreover there is good evidence that antibiotic treatment of asymptomatic bacteriuria reduces the risk of both these outcomes. Consequently all pregnant women should be screened in the first trimester of pregnancy and women with bacteriuria should be treated.

Asymptomatic bacteriuria should not be treated with antibiotics in any other people. Placebo controlled trials have failed to show convincing benefit in patients with diabetes, in institutionalized elderly men or women, or in those with long-term indwelling catheters, whereas the same trials did show increased risk of adverse events in the treated patients, including colonization with antibiotic-resistant bacteria.

Choice of agent

Lower urinary tract infection

In lower urinary tract infection seen in general practice, over 90% of patients become asymptomatic after a few days' appropriate antibiotic therapy and remain free from bacteriuria for several weeks or more. Most current practice guidelines recommend empirical treatment with a 'best guess' antibiotic selected based on knowledge of likely pathogens and local resistance patterns. In domiciliary practice *Escherichia coli* predominates and most will be fully sensitive to all the commonly used antimicrobials listed in Table 20.1. However, ampicillin-resistant organisms are now sufficiently common for this drug to be abandoned in favour of trimethoprim or one of the other oral agents. The use of co-trimoxazole is not recommended in the treatment of urinary infection, since the sulphonamide component plays an insignificant role and trimethoprim alone is less toxic.

Two agents, nitrofurantoin and nalidixic acid, achieve adequate concentrations only in urine and are exclusively used in lower urinary tract infection. Nitrofurantoin has the distinct advantage of being unrelated to other antibiotics. In contrast nalidixic acid is a quinolone and is likely to select for bacteria that are resistant to fluoroquinolones such as ciprofloxacin. For that reason nitrofurantoin is usually recommended as the preferred alternative to trimethoprim for lower urinary tract infection.

For bacteria that are resistant to nitrofurantoin and trimethoprim or for patients who cannot tolerate these drugs there is a range of alternative oral agents, including oral cephalosporins, co-amoxiclav, fluoroquinolones, and pivmecillinam. The reason that these drugs are not used first line is that they are no more effective than nitrofurantoin or trimethoprim and should be reserved for patients in whom these first line agents are ineffective or contraindicated.

Upper urinary tract infection

Upper urinary tract infection can be accompanied by bacteraemia, making it a life-threatening infection. However, infection should respond to effective antibiotic treatment in 90% of patients.

Nitrofurantoin is not an effective treatment for upper urinary tract infection because it does not achieve effective concentrations in the blood. Resistance to trimethoprim is too common to recommend this drug for empirical treatment of a life-threatening infection. Consequently, empirical treatment should be with a broad-spectrum antibiotic such as co-amoxiclav or ciprofloxacin.

Because of the potentially serious consequences of upper urinary tract infections it is recommended that urine cultures should be obtained before starting antibiotic treatment in all patients. This is because community-acquired infection can be caused by pathogens that are resistant to either co-amoxiclav, ciprofloxacin or any of the other oral antibiotics used in general practice and this is not an acceptable risk with a life-threatening infection.

Therapeutic regimens

In the special circumstances of urinary infection, unlike those in other parts of the body, the drugs used are often preferentially excreted into the urine and may attain very high concentrations there, sometimes for long periods. Moreover, in the treatment of lower urinary tract infection (in contrast to pyelonephritis or infections complicating urinary tract abnormalities) antibacterial drugs are generally needed only to tip the balance in favour of normal clearance mechanisms. Several studies have shown that much-curtailed regimens, lasting 1–3 days, are as successful as prolonged therapy in curing acute urinary infections. Indeed, longer courses are wasteful of resources especially since many patients, wiser than their doctors, abandon treatment once the symptoms abate.

Short-course treatment has an additional potential benefit in serving to identify those few patients (the ones who fail short-course therapy) who are likely to require more extensive urological investigation. Most current guidelines recommend 3 days' treatment with trimethoprim for uncompli-cated lower urinary tract infection but there is less certainty about nitrofurantoin. UK guidelines recommend 3 days' therapy but guidelines in other countries recommend treatment for 5 or 7 days.

Management of common clinical problems

Acute symptomatic infections in children

Diagnosis of symptomatic urinary tract infection is rarely straightforward, especially in younger children. They may present with generalized symptoms (fever, vomiting, general malaise) rather than with symptoms in the urinary tract. Consequently, clinically, suspicion should be confirmed by urine culture. If it is difficult to obtain a high-quality clean catch midstream specimen of urine then diagnosis may have to rely on obtaining urine by catheterization or suprapubic needle aspirate. In a child with a low clinical suspicion of urinary tract infection in whom these tests are considered unnecessarily invasive urine dipstick testing can be used, followed by culture of urine only if the dipstick results suggest bacteriuria. However, false negative dipstick tests do occur.

Acute symptomatic infections in adult women

Clinical diagnosis of lower urinary tract infection is reliable in young adult women who have dysuria and frequency but no history of vaginal discharge. Neither dipstick tests nor urine culture are necessary to confirm the diagnosis and empiric antibiotic treatment (3 days of trimethoprim or nitrofurantoin) should be given on the basis of these symptoms alone. If the symptoms are less clear-cut (e.g. the patient has frequency or dysuria but not both) then urine dipstick testing should be done. If this is positive then 3 days of trimethoprim or nitrofurantoin should be given, but if it is negative bacteriuria should be confirmed with culture before treatment is given.

If the woman has symptoms of upper tract infection (loin pain or systemic inflammatory response) then a urine culture should be taken before empiric treatment is started in order to identify resistant bacteria. Empiric treatment should be with co-amoxiclav, pivmecillinam, or a fluoroquinolone for 7 days.

Urinary tract infection is difficult to diagnose in older women because it is more likely to present with vague, generalized symptoms. Moreover the prevalence of asymptomatic bacteriuria increases steadily with age and with increasing co-morbidity. Over 50% of institutionalized elderly women have asymptomatic bacteriuria all of the time. The decision to give antibiotic treatment should be based on clinical diagnosis of infection, supported by acute local or systemic symptoms of inflammation. Smelly urine just means that the patient has bacteriuria, which is not unusual and does not require antibiotic treatment.

Recurrent symptomatic infections in women

Recurrent urinary tract infection in healthy non-pregnant women is defined as three or more episodes during a 12-month period. Antibiotics can be used to reduce the frequency of recurrent infection in two ways. A single dose of either trimethoprim or nitrofurantoin taken at night reduces the risk of symptomatic infection to about one-fifth of the risk with no treatment. However, the risk of recurrent urinary infection returns to pretreatment levels as soon as treatment is stopped. An alternative, equally effective strategy for women with infection associated with sexual intercourse is to take a single postcoital dose of antibiotic. Prophylactic antibiotics for recurrent infection have side effects (oral or vaginal candidiasis and gastrointestinal symptoms) but infection by bacteria resistant to the prophylactic antibiotic does not appear to be a significant risk.

Organism	Site	Disease	Treatment	Comments
Norovirus	Small bowel[b]	'Winter vomiting disease'	None	Outbreaks occur
Rotavirus	Small bowel[b]	Diarrhoea	None	Outbreaks occur
Salmonella enterica serotypes Typhi and Paratyphi	Extra-intestinal	Enteric fever	Ciprofloxacin, chloramphenicol or co-trimoxazole	Antibiotic treatment mandatory; resistance occurs
Other salmonellae	Small bowel[b]	Diarrhoea	None	Ciprofloxacin in systemic infection
Shigella sonnei	Large bowel[b]	Sonnei dysentery	None	Usually self-limiting
Other shigellae	Large bowel[b]	Bacillary dysentery	Ciprofloxacin; co-trimoxazole	Antibiotics in severe cases only
Staphylococcus aureus	Small bowel	Food poisoning (vomiting)	None	Due to enterotoxin
Vibrio cholerae	Small bowel	Cholera	Doxycycline; ciprofloxacin	Fluid replacement essential
Yersinia enterocolitica	Small bowel	Mesenteric adenitis/ileitis	Ciprofloxacin, co-trimoxazole	Antibiotics in severe cases only

[a] Other serotypes are sometimes involved.

[b] Mucosal invasion.

[c] Routine use not recommended.

to fluid and electrolyte replacement therapy. The duration of diarrhoea is decreased and the volume of stool is reduced by almost half by the use of an oral tetracycline such as doxycycline, prescribed as a single dose of 300 mg in adults. Resistance to tetracyclines is, unfortunately, increasing. Alternatives include co-trimoxazole, azithromycin, or ciprofloxacin (although fluoroquinolone resistant strains have emerged in India). The vibrio is eliminated from the bowel and toxin production ceases rapidly. The carrier state does not occur but transmission from dead bodies has been reported.

Campylobacter infection

Campylobacter jejuni (or occasionally *Campylobacter coli*) is among the commonest causes of sporadic acute gastrointestinal infection throughout the world. The organism produces infection in all age groups, but most frequently in young adults and pre-school children. Epidemics have occurred involving several thousand people following the ingestion of contaminated milk or water supplies. Campylobacters cause infection in domestic and farm animals, poultry and wild birds, and hence there are many opportunities for spread to humans. Importantly, campylobacter infection is occasionally complicated by the development of Guillain–Barré syndrome or reactive arthritis.

Campylobacter gastroenteritis generally lasts for a few days, but may occasionally be more protracted with marked abdominal symptoms of colicky pain and tenderness as well as profuse diarrhoea. Acute appendicitis may be mimicked. Attacks are self-limiting and managed mainly by increasing the oral fluid intake. Although campylobacter infection is common, fatalities are rare. Excretion ceases soon after clinical recovery. Antibiotic therapy is not beneficial in most cases. Cases with severe or prolonged symptoms may benefit from oral therapy with erythromycin or a fluoroquinolone such as ciprofloxacin. However, the prevalence of resistance to these agents has increased, probably related to their use in animal husbandry.

Helicobacter infection

Helicobacter pylori is an important cause of chronic gastritis and gastroduodenal ulceration. It is also likely to be responsible for some cases of gastric carcinoma. Treatment of *H. pylori* infection usually involves 7 days' therapy with two antibiotics (various combinations of clarithromycin, metronidazole and amoxicillin are often used) together with a proton pump inhibitor such as omeprazole. Approximately 10% of patients fail treatment.

There is evidence for increasing antibiotic resistance among *H. pylori* strains, particularly in individuals who have previously received metronidazole. Resistance to metronidazole occurs in approximately 50% of infected individuals in many European countries with levels of up to 90% in developing countries. Resistance to clarithromycin is currently below 10% in many European countries, but rates may be increasing. Pretreatment resistance to clarithromycin can reduce the effectiveness of therapy by about 50%. Resistance to amoxicillin or tetracycline is presently uncommon.

Salmonellosis

Intestinal salmonellosis

Gastrointestinal salmonellosis is second only to campylobacter as a bacterial cause of community acquired gastrointestinal infection; several thousand cases are reported annually in the UK. There are more than 2400 different serotypes of *Salmonella enterica*, although relatively few regularly cause human disease. Some common serotypes are Typhimurium, Enteritidis, Hadar, and Virchow. Frozen poultry and eggs are a common source of infection, which is easily transmitted among battery hens and during the evisceration of carcasses. Measures to control infection in chickens have markedly reduced the incidence of salmonella infection in the UK.

Illness is commonly associated with systemic features of fever and malaise, in addition to the gastrointestinal symptoms. Bloodstream invasion may occur following mucosal penetration. Bloodstream infection complicating salmonella gastroenteritis is more likely in the very young and the elderly, and in those with underlying diseases such as alcoholism, cirrhosis, and AIDS. Achlorhydria from pernicious anaemia, atrophic gastritis, gastrectomy, or therapy with H_2-receptor antagonists or proton pump inhibitor enhances the risk of salmonellosis by eliminating the protection afforded by the normal gastric acid so that the number of bacteria needed to be ingested to cause infection is reduced.

Treatment of acute gastrointestinal salmonellosis is essentially directed at the replacement of any lost fluid or electrolytes, either by mouth or intravenously. Antibiotics are usually unnecessary unless there is secondary bloodstream invasion, since they do not reduce the duration of illness. Antibiotic treatment may also be associated with increased incidence of carriage of salmonellae. For severe or invasive infections fluoroquinolones are useful, although resistance is becoming more common. Co-trimoxazole or a cephalosporin, such as ceftriaxone, provide alternative choices. The emergence of multiresistant strains, some with transferable genes, compromises treatment choices in some parts of the world. Local epidemiological surveillance data can help guide empirical therapy.

Enteric (typhoid and paratyphoid) fever

Enteric fever is caused by *Salmonella enterica* serotypes Typhi or Paratyphi A, B, or C. This is primarily a septicaemic illness acquired by ingestion of the bacterium followed by mucosal invasion. The pathogen gains access to the lymphatics and blood from where it infects the liver and other parts of the reticuloendothelial system. The bowel is also involved since the lymphoid tissue in Peyer's patches is inflamed and often ulcerates. Notably, constipation is more common than diarrhoea. Perforation and peritonitis are not uncommon in untreated cases. Enteric fever is potentially fatal and, unlike gastrointestinal salmonellosis, should always be treated with antibiotics. The bacteria are often located intracellularly and drugs active in vitro may not evoke a satisfactory clinical response.

The antibiotic of choice for enteric fever is ciprofloxacin, which produces the most rapid resolution of fever and best cure rates. Treatment must be continued for 2 weeks and, even so, relapse may occur. Relapses should be treated for a further 2 weeks. Resistance to fluoroquinolones has emerged. Alternative agents with variable activity include chloramphenicol, co-trimoxazole, and high-dose amoxicillin. For multiresistant strains cephalosporins such as ceftriaxone or cefixime (which can be given orally) have proved useful. Because of the threat of multiresistant strains, the susceptibility of clinical isolates should be tested in the laboratory whenever possible. In severe infection steroids given in the first 48 h may be beneficial.

Although typhoid vaccines are available they are not recommended for international travel unless there is a high risk of exposure.

Salmonella carriage

Salmonellae may be excreted in faeces for several weeks after clinical recovery. If this continues for more than 3 months it is likely that the patient will become a persistent carrier. Chronic carriage is uncommon (<5%) but more frequent in infants and in people with biliary disease (including bile stones) or schistosomal bladder infection. The chronic carrier is normally harmless to the individual, but may be a threat to the household and the community if lapses in personal hygiene cause contamination of food or water supplies. Importantly, humans are the only natural host for *Salmonella* Typhi and so it is important to identify and treat carriers as a public health control measure. Chronic excretion precludes employment as a food handler. Ciprofloxacin is the preferred treatment for carriers; alternatively, prolonged high-dosage ampicillin may be curative.

Shigellosis

Shigellosis in its most severe form is characterized by profuse diarrhoea with blood and pus; i.e. classic bacillary dysentery. Infection is more common in underdeveloped countries where sanitation and levels of hygiene are low. In developed countries shigellosis (usually caused by *Sh. sonnei*) occurs particularly among young children in nurseries and schools, and also in long-stay institutions such as prisons and psychiatric hospitals. The spectrum of illness ranges from mild diarrhoea to a fulminating attack of dysentery. The more severe forms of disease are associated with *Shigella dysenteriae*, whereas milder symptoms are caused by *Sh. sonnei*. *Shigella flexneri* and *Shigella boydii* tend to produce disease of intermediate severity. *Shigella* spp. are among the most virulent gastrointestinal pathogens, requiring only few bacteria to produce disease. The bacteria multiply in the small bowel with subsequent invasion of the mucosa of the terminal ileum and colon. The intense inflammatory response produces a hyperaemic bowel which readily bleeds, although bloodstream invasion is uncommon. Some strains, notably *Sh. dysenteriae*, produce an enterotoxin (Shiga toxin) that stimulates fluid secretion in the small bowel, so that watery diarrhoea may precede frank dysentery. Occasionally, haemolytic uraemic syndrome (see below) occurs.

Treatment of shigellosis is dependent on the severity of the diarrhoea and blood loss. Mild attacks, including most *Sh. sonnei* cases, may be managed by oral rehydration with glucose-salts solution. More severe cases may require admission to hospital and intravenous fluids. In severe shigellosis there is a definite place for antibiotic therapy. In addition treatment is sometimes used to shorten symptoms and bacterial excretion, particularly in outbreaks. Three days of treatment with oral ciprofloxacin, co-trimoxazole, ampicillin, or tetracycline have been widely used. However, resistance to each of these agents occurs, and laboratory testing of susceptibility is important.

Escherichia coli

Distinct types of *Esch. coli* cause a wide spectrum of gastrointestinal infection.

- **Enterotoxigenic *Esch. coli*** cause most cases of traveller's diarrhoea. The toxins have many similarities to cholera toxin and the pathophysiology of the illness is similar, though fatalities are uncommon.

- **Enteropathogenic *Esch. coli*** is now largely confined to developing countries where it remains a leading cause of severe diarrhoea in the very young.

- **Entero-invasive Esch. coli** can produce severe invasive (dysentery-like) infection of the bowel, but are fortunately uncommon.

- **Enterohaemorrhagic Esch. coli** (principally *Esch. coli* O157) produce a shiga-like toxin. In addition to haemorrhagic colitis these strains can cause renal impairment and haemolysis (haemolytic uraemic syndrome); this develops in approximately 5% of affected children during outbreaks.

- **Entero-aggregative Esch. coli** show characteristic patterns of adherence to epithelial cells.

Antimicrobial therapy is usually unnecessary in the treatment of gastro-intestinal infections with *Esch. coli*. Indeed, in haemolytic uraemic syndrome antibiotic administration is contraindicated because of the chance of exacerbating symptoms, presumably because of antibiotic-mediated bacterial cell lysis and toxin release.

The use of antibiotics to prevent traveller's diarrhoea is not recommended because of the possibility of encouraging the emergence of multiresistant strains, the risk of side effects, and the generally mild nature of the infection. If diarrhoea develops fluoroquinolones can alleviate symptoms within 24 h. If the importance of the trip warrants the use of prophylaxis, fluoroquinolones, tetracyclines, or co-trimoxazole appear to be effective.

Yersiniosis

Infection with *Yersinia enterocolitica* may produce mesenteric adenitis, terminal ileitis, and acute diarrhoea. Erythema nodosum and a reactive arthritis may complicate such infections. The illness is usually self-limiting and, unless complicated by extra-gastrointestinal symptoms, is infrequently suspected. Ciprofloxacin, co-trimoxazole, or tetracycline are effective in severe cases.

Intestinal parasites

Some protozoa and helminths may cause symptoms ranging from mild diarrhoea to severe dysentery. These are considered in Chapters 5 and 30.

Antibiotic-associated diarrhoea

The use of antimicrobial agents is sometimes complicated by diarrhoea. This is most often due to a direct effect on gut motility or the bowel mucosa. However, about 20% of cases are caused by toxin producing strains of *Clostridium difficile*. *C. difficile* may have a competitive advantage over the normal gut flora following antibiotic exposure, notably in the elderly.

inflammation might act as a beneficial adjunct to antimicrobial therapy in septic patients.

Monoclonal antibodies against lipid A of Gram-negative bacteria and against various cytokines, such as interleukin-1 and tumour necrosis factor, have been subjected to therapeutic trial. To date, none has shown clinical benefit. Most recently, recombinant activated Protein C (drotrecogin alfa) has shown some benefit in reducing mortality in selected patients with septic shock and organ dysfunction. The pathophysiology of sepsis is extremely complex, suggesting that no single strategy is likely to prove effective in all patients.

Infective endocarditis

Endocarditis is inflammation of the endocardial surface of the heart. When caused by micro-organisms it is known as 'infective' endocarditis, and may be caused by bacteria including, rickettsiae, chlamydiae, and also fungi. Endocarditis usually affects the heart valves but may involve the adjacent endocardium. The terms acute and subacute endocarditis originated in the pre-antibiotic era when all patients with endocarditis died. Those who died in less than 6 weeks due to infection of normal valves by virulent organisms such as *Staph. aureus*, *Str. pneumoniae*, or *N. gonorrhoeae* were said to have acute bacterial endocarditis. In contrast, those who suffered a more indolent course due to infection of abnormal valves by relatively avirulent organisms (e.g. viridans streptococci), died much later and were said to have subacute bacterial endocarditis.

Nowadays, most patients with infective endocarditis are cured provided the diagnosis is made, and treatment with appropriate antibiotics begun sufficiently early. It is also more useful to classify endocarditis according to the infecting organism and the underlying site of infection (e.g. *Staph. aureus* tricuspid endocarditis). In addition, distinguishing native from prosthetic valve infection is also important. These definitions are of value in predicting the probable course of the disease and also have therapeutic implications with regard to the antibiotic regimen to be used.

Epidemiology

Infective endocarditis affects about 2000 people per year in England and Wales and has a mortality of 15–30%. In recent years the spectrum of recognized underlying cardiac lesions in endocarditis in adults has changed as a result of a decline in rheumatic heart disease (in the developed world), the increase of endocarditis complicating degenerative heart disease and improvement in diagnostic techniques (echocardiography). The following trends have been noted:

* The mean age of the patient has increased; it is now over 50 years of age for the following reasons:
    * people with congenital heart disease or rheumatic heart disease survive longer because of advances in medical and surgical expertise to correct valve dysfunction;
    * increased life expectancy is associated with a raised incidence of degenerative valve disease; almost 30% of elderly patients who develop endocarditis do not have a pre-existing cardiac condition. Minor degenerative changes produce valvular lesions that serve as a nidus for infection;
    * infectious complications of genitourinary and gastrointestinal disease predispose to bacteraemia in elderly people.
* Acute *Staph. aureus* endocarditis is an important complication of intravenous drug-abusers.
* Mitral valve prolapse with regurgitation predisposes to endocarditis and is now recognized more frequently.
* Prosthetic valve endocarditis has increased in proportion to cardiac valve surgery.
* The 'classic' physical signs of subacute bacterial endocarditis are seen in fewer patients as a result of earlier diagnosis.

Pathogenesis

Infective endocarditis is the consequence of several events (Fig. 22.1):

* haemodynamic or disease associated damage to the endothelial surface of the valve;
* deposition of platelets and fibrin on the edges of the valve, initially resulting in the formation of sterile or non-bacterial thrombotic vegetation;
* colonization by micro-organisms transiently circulating in the blood to produce an infected vegetation.

Transient bacteraemia is common. A wide variety of trivial events (e.g. chewing and tooth-brushing) can induce bacteraemia with oral streptococci. Some 85% of cases of streptococcal endocarditis cannot be related to any medical or dental procedure. To cause endocarditis, organisms must also be

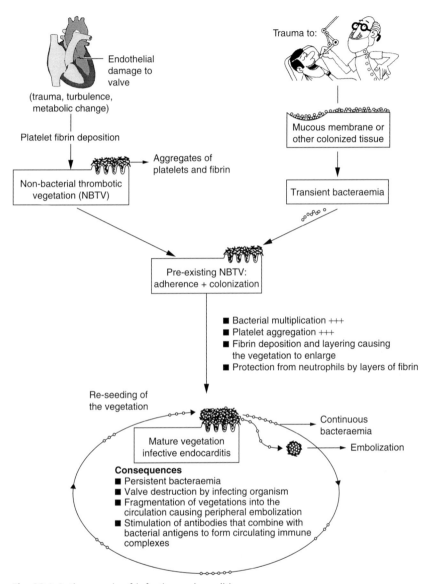

Fig. 22.1 Pathogenesis of infective endocarditis.

able to survive natural complement-mediated serum bactericidal activity and adhere to thrombotic vegetations. Certain streptococci produce extracellular dextran, which promotes adherence to fibrin–platelet vegetations. These strains cause endocarditis more frequently than non-dextran producing streptococci. However, organisms such as enterococci and *Staph. aureus* that do not produce dextran are also important causes of endocarditis. In these cases host proteins such as fibronectin and fibrinogen may mediate adherence.

Once colonization occurs there is rapid deposition of additional layers of platelets and fibrin over and around the growing colonies, causing the vegetation to enlarge. Within 24–48 h marked proliferation of bacteria occurs, leading to dense populations of organisms (10^9–10^{10} bacteria/g tissue). Micro-organisms deep within the vegetations are often metabolically inactive, whereas the more superficial ones proliferate and are shed continuously into the bloodstream. Fresh vegetations are composed of colonies of micro-organisms in a fibrin–platelet matrix with very few leucocytes.

Aetiological agents

Any organism can cause infective endocarditis, but streptococci and staphylococci account for more than 90% of culture-positive cases. However, the frequency with which various organisms are involved differs not only for the type of valve that is infected (native or prosthetic) but also with the causative event (e.g. dental manipulation, intravenous drug abuse, or a hospital-acquired infection) (Table 22.3).

Native-valve endocarditis

Streptococci

Streptococci account for about 65% of all cases of native valve endocarditis. Most common of all are the 'viridans streptococci', which include *Streptococcus mitis*, *Str. sanguis*, *Str. mutans*, the *Str. milleri* group, and *Str. salivarius*, which are mouth commensals; most are highly sensitive to penicillin and cause infections primarily on abnormal heart valves. *Str. bovis* is an important cause of endocarditis in elderly people and is frequently associated with bowel pathology, notably colonic polyps and carcinoma. Recovery of this organism should prompt investigation for colonic disease.

Enterococci are gut streptococci and cause 10% of cases. Haemolytic streptococci of Lancefield groups B and G are occasionally incriminated in endocarditis. Diabetic patients are particularly at risk of group B infections.

Staphylococci

Staphylococci account for 25% of cases of native valve endocarditis, but over 90% is due to *Staph. aureus*, which is the leading cause of acute endocarditis. The course is frequently fulminant with widespread metastatic abscesses and death in about 40% of cases. The organism can attack normal or damaged valves and cause rapid destruction of the affected valves. Surgery is often

Aminoglycoside assays

When aminoglycosides (usually gentamicin) are used to treat endocarditis, a serum concentration lower than that considered therapeutic for Gram-negative infections is adequate, thus lessening the potential for toxicity. Patients with normal renal function should receive a loading dose appropriate to the age and body weight, followed by a maintenance dose. The serum concentration should be periodically monitored and the dose adjusted accordingly (a pre-dose concentration <1.0 mg/l; post-dose 4–5 mg/l is adequate).

Specific antimicrobial regimens

Streptococci

Isolates highly sensitive to penicillin (MIC <0.1 mg/l)
This includes most viridans streptococci, *Str. bovis*, and other streptococci. Viridans streptococci are highly sensitive to penicillin and a 99% cure rate can be achieved with a 4-week regimen of benzylpenicillin alone. Such a regimen is recommended for the treatment of uncomplicated native valve endocarditis in elderly patients, or those with impaired renal function, in whom aminoglycosides are best avoided.

For uncomplicated native valve endocarditis it is common practice in the UK to give 2 weeks of combination therapy with high-dose benzylpenicillin together with an aminoglycoside and then to consider oral amoxicillin for the last 2 weeks if patient compliance can be guaranteed. Patients with prosthetic valve endocarditis should be treated for longer to ensure cure; 6 weeks is recommended.

Isolates relatively resistant to penicillin (MIC 0.1–0.5 mg/l)
This category includes some viridans streptococci such as the 'nutritionally variant' streptococci. Viridans streptococci that are relatively resistant to penicillin are increasingly encountered. The relapse rate in endocarditis caused by 'nutritionally variant' streptococci is high, even when 2 weeks of combination therapy is followed by 2 further weeks of benzylpenicillin. Endocarditis caused by such strains or other streptococci that are relatively resistant to penicillin is best treated with high-dose benzylpenicillin and gentamicin for 4 weeks, with appropriate monitoring of serum gentamicin levels.

Isolates resistant to penicillin (MIC >0.5 mg/l)
Examples are *Enterococcus faecalis*, *Ent. faecium*, and other streptococci. Enterococcal endocarditis is the third most common type of endocarditis

and is among the most difficult to treat. Mortality is about 20% and relapses are not uncommon. Although penicillin, ampicillin, and vancomycin inhibit the growth of enterococci they are not bactericidal for most strains, and therapy with these agents alone results in a high relapse rate. For a bactericidal effect, it is usually necessary to add an aminoglycoside; this results in marked enhancement of killing. A combination of penicillin or ampicillin with an aminoglycoside is the treatment of choice for enterococcal endocarditis; gentamicin is the preferred aminoglycoside. High-level resistance to gentamicin among enterococci is becoming more common and in-vitro testing (with a disc containing 100 mg of gentamicin) should be a routine procedure in all isolates of enterococci.

Ent. faecium is generally more resistant to β-lactam antibiotics than *Ent. faecalis*; β-lactamase-producing *Ent. faecalis* strains have also been reported. Such patients are best treated with vancomycin and gentamicin. Enterococci are uniformly resistant to all cephalosporins. Patients with enterococcal endocarditis should receive at least 4–6 weeks of combination therapy.

Staphylococci

Staphylococcus aureus

In about one-third of patients with *Staph. aureus* endocarditis there is no evidence of pre-existing valvular heart disease. The infection results in rapid and severe valvular destruction and a mortality of about 40% even with appropriate treatment.

Patients over 50 years of age with *Staph. aureus* endocarditis secondary to infected intravascular devices have the highest mortality rate. Many require surgery to replace the infected valve, because of valvular dysfunction, dehiscence, and myocardial abscesses. In contrast, *Staph. aureus* endocarditis involving the tricuspid valve in intravenous drug abusers is much easier to cure and carries a mortality below 10%.

Since the vast majority of *Staph. aureus* strains produce a β-lactamase that destroys penicillin, the initial choice is a penicillinase-stable penicillin such as flucloxacillin. However, the choice and duration of treatment with a synergistic agent (e.g. gentamicin) remains controversial. Flucloxacillin plus gentamicin is associated with a more rapid clearance of bacteraemia. In the UK, low-dose gentamicin is widely used with flucloxacillin for both native valve and prosthetic valve endocarditis, at least for the first 2 weeks of therapy.

In selected patients, such as an intravenous drug abuser with a right-sided endocarditis, or a patient with uncomplicated native valve endocarditis, who has responded fully to 2 weeks of combination therapy, oral

Table 22.4 Recommended antibiotic treatment regimens for streptococcal endocarditis

Organism	Treatment of choice	Suggested adult dosage/interval/route	Comments
(a) Highly sensitive to penicillin (MIC <0.1 mg/l) Viridans streptococci Str. bovis Other streptococci	Benzylpenicillin (4 weeks) Gentamicin (weeks 1–2)	1.2 g/4 h/i.v.	**Native valve endocarditis (NVE):** Consider benzylpenicillin alone for 4 weeks for elderly people or those at risk of renal problems Consider change to oral amoxicillin (1 g/6 h) after 2 weeks combination therapy In uncomplicated infections 2 weeks combination therapy may be adequate **Prosthetic valve endocarditis (PVE):** Gentamicin included for at least 2 weeks, then benzylpenicillin for a further 4 weeks; or oral amoxicillin (1 g/6 h) after 4 weeks benzylpenicillin (ceftriaxone/vancomycin[a])
(b) Relatively resistant to penicillin (MIC 0.1–0.5 mg/l) Nutritionally variant or viridans streptococci	Benzylpenicillin (4 weeks) Gentamicin (4 weeks)	1.2 g/4 h/i.v.	The relapse rate is high; combination therapy may be prolonged for 4 weeks
(c) Resistant to penicillin (MIC >0.5 mg/l) Enterococci Viridans streptococci	Ampicillin (4 weeks) Gentamicin (4 weeks)	2 g/4 h/ i.v.	Ampicillin more active than benzylpenicillin for enterococci. To avoid relapse, prolong combination therapy for 6 weeks if: (1) PVE; (2) symptoms for >3 months; (3) mitral valve involved; (4) relapse of enterococcal endocarditis (vancomycin[a])

[a]Alternative drugs if patient is allergic to penicillin.

PVE, prosthetic valve endocarditis.

Table 22.5 Recommended antibiotic treatment regimens for staphylococcal endocarditis

Organism	Treatment of choice	Suggested adult dosage/interval/route	Comments
Staph. aureus	Flucloxacillin (4 weeks) Gentamicin (weeks 1–2)	3 g/6 h/i.v.	In selected patients consider oral flucloxacillin after 2 weeks (see text) In complicated or PVE flucloxacillin may be prolonged for 6 weeks; consider adding rifampicin (300–600 mg b.d. oral). Use vancomycin 1 g/12 h/i.v. for methicillin-resistant strains, or if allergic to penicillin. Surgery often required
Staph. epidermidis	Vancomycin (6 weeks) Rifampicin (6 weeks) Gentamicin (weeks 1–3)	1 g/12 h/i.v. 300–600 mg/12 h/oral	Most strains resistant to flucloxacillin; use rifampicin and gentamicin if susceptible; prolong vancomycin and rifampicin for 6 weeks; surgery often required

PVE, prosthetic valve endocarditis.

flucloxacillin may be considered for the remaining 2 weeks of therapy. The remaining patients should receive high-dose flucloxacillin intravenously for at least 4 weeks.

If the patient is allergic to penicillin or the *Staph. aureus* is multiresistant, then vancomycin should be used. Rifampicin, a very potent antistaphylococcal agent, should be added in difficult cases but is never used alone, owing to the emergence of resistance.

Staphylococcus epidermidis

This organism rarely infects a native valve, but is a common cause of both early and late onset prosthetic valve endocarditis. It is difficult to cure with antibiotics alone, and surgery is often required, particularly in patients with early-onset endocarditis. Isolates are frequently resistant to flucloxacillin, which must not be used unless the isolate is confirmed to be sensitive. Therapy must therefore be started with vancomycin and rifampicin. Gentamicin may be added for the first 2–3 weeks, if the strain is sensitive. Frequent monitoring of gentamicin levels is mandatory to minimize the risk of toxicity. If the organism is indeed sensitive to flucloxacillin then vancomycin is stopped and flucloxacillin and rifampicin are continued.

Table 23.1 Most likely bacterial causes and antibacterial treatment for common skin infections

Clinical diagnosis	Most likely causes	Antibacterial treatment
Impetigo	*Str. pyogenes*	Topical: fusidic acid or mupirocin; reserve for patients with a limited number of lesions
	Staph. aureus	Systemic: antistaphylococcal penicillin (e.g. flucloxacillin), clindamycin or a tetracycline
Pustules, furuncles and carbuncles	*Staph. aureus*	Small lesions: no treatment is required in most cases
		Larger lesions: incision and drainage. Antibiotics required only if there are signs of spreading cellulitis or systemic inflammation
		Recurrent lesions: topical mupirocin to the nose for the first 5 days of each month. If this fails try clindamycin 150 mg once daily dose for 3 months
Uncomplicated cellulitis and erysipelas	*Str. pyogenes*	Antistaphylococcal penicillin (e.g. flucloxacillin),
	Staph. aureus	Clindamycin or a tetracycline
Necrotizing fasciitis	*Str. pyogenes* *Staph. aureus* Gram-negative aerobic bacteria Anaerobic bacteria	Clindamycin plus a fluoroquinolone
Animal bites	Bacteria from the animal's normal mouth flora (e.g. *Pasteurella multocida*)	Co-amoxiclav. For penicillin allergic patients doxycycline plus metronidazole
Human bites	Mixed aerobic and anaerobic mouth flora	Co-amoxiclav. For penicillin allergic patients clindamycin plus a fluoroquinolone
Diabetic foot infections	*Str. pyogenes* *Staph. aureus* Gram-negative aerobic bacteria Anaerobic bacteria	Co-amoxiclav. For penicillin allergic patients clindamycin + a fluoroquinolone

and normal skin, with a palpable lesion that is raised above the level of the normal skin. Cellulitis may be caused by *Str. pyogenes* or *Staph. aureus,* whereas erysipelas is almost always caused by *Str. pyogenes.* Erysipelas usually occurs on the face or on the legs, whereas cellulitis can occur anywhere on the body although it is commonest on the legs. Both types of lesion are usually preceded by a break in the skin. Methicillin-resistant *Staph. aureus* (MRSA) is increasingly incriminated in community-acquired cellulitis in some countries.

Signs of spreading infection include extension of the line of demarcation, lymphangitis (infection spreading up the lymph vessels with a characteristic thin streak of erythema running up to a lymph node), and painful tender lymph nodes distal to the lesion. Systemic inflammatory response means that the patient has sepsis and is at risk of progressing to severe sepsis or septic shock (see p. 310). Blood cultures should be taken from patients with sepsis arising from cellulitis, as about 50% are positive.

Both cellulitis and erysipelas can be treated with an antistaphylococcal penicillin. In theory erysipelas could be treated with penicillin V, but it is not worth taking the risk that the cause may be *Staph. aureus.* There is a belief that an antistaphylococcal penicillin should be combined with benzylpenicillin or penicillin V, since the latter are much more active against *Str. pyogenes.* However, provided antistaphylococcal penicillins are given in adequate dosage they are just as effective alone.

Prevention of recurrent cellulitis requires enhancement of host defences by preventing breaks in the skin (e.g. dry thoroughly between the toes after washing), or wearing compression stockings to reduce oedema. If these measures fail then long-term prophylactic antibiotics are unfortunately not usually effective. It is preferable to give the patient a course of antibiotics to start as soon as symptoms begin.

Necrotizing skin and soft tissue infections

These are rapidly spreading and life-threatening forms of cellulitis that involve the deeper fascial and/or muscle compartments in addition to skin and subcutaneous tissue. Infection usually arises following a break in the skin after trauma or elective surgery. Most cases are caused by *Str. pyogenes* either alone or in combination with other bacteria, including *Staph. aureus,* coliform bacilli, and anaerobes. Many variations of nectrotizing skin and soft tissue infections have been described according to the tissues involved, the anatomical site of the infection and the microbial causes but the basic principles of management are the same. The key is early distinction between a cellulitis that will respond to antibacterial treatment and a deeper necrotizing infection that is likely to require surgical debridement as well. The following clinical features indicate the possibility of necrotizing infection:

- severe, constant pain that is disproportionate to the visible inflammation in the skin;
- bullae on the skin, which occur because of occlusion of deep blood vessels that cross the fascia or muscle compartments;
- skin necrosis or bruising;
- gas in the soft tissues detected by palpation or imaging;
- oedema that extends beyond the margin of erythema;
- cutaneous anaesthesia;
- systemic toxicity, manifested by signs of severe sepsis (p. 185);
- rapid spread of infection despite appropriate antibiotic therapy.

Blood cultures are often positive and streptococci can also be isolated from the bullous lesions. The management of these rare conditions is primarily surgical, with radical debridement of all necrotic tissue, intensive life-support therapy, and the treatment of shock. Antimicrobial therapy must be directed against aerobic Gram-positive and Gram-negative bacteria and against anaerobic bacteria until the results of cultures are available. Clindamycin is active against aerobic Gram-positive and anaerobic pathogens, it also suppresses toxin production by group A streptococci and may be superior to penicillins for these infections. A fluoroquinolone should be added initially to treat Gram-negative aerobic pathogens.

Gas gangrene

Gas gangrene (clostridial myositis) is a life-threatening, invasive infection that can be caused by several species of *Clostridium*, principally *C. perfringens*. These bacteria are part of the normal intestinal flora of man and animals, and clostridial spores are common in soil. Gas gangrene develops when impaired blood supply, tissue necrosis, or the presence of foreign bodies produce a low oxygen tension in the tissues and thus create conditions in which the spores can germinate. Extensive soft-tissue injury contaminated with soil or dirt carries an increased risk of gas gangrene. Gas gangrene may rarely complicate surgical wounds, particularly after intestinal or biliary surgery, or be a complication of septic abortion. Clostridial anaerobic cellulitis occurs under similar circumstances, but exploration of the wound usually reveals that the muscle is spared.

A clinical diagnosis is made on the basis of palpable (crepitus) or radiological signs of a spreading, gas-producing infection in a toxic patient with the above risk factors. Immediate and extensive surgical excision of all involved tissues and the removal of any foreign body are essential, and may mean hysterectomy (after septic abortion), excision of subcutaneous tissue and muscle of the abdominal wall, or even amputation of a limb. Parenteral benzylpenicillin should also be given promptly in high dosage. For patients allergic to penicillin, metronidazole may be used. Despite these desperate and mutilating measures, the mortality remains high.

Cellulitis following animal or human bites

Infections following animal bites are polymicrobial, often include anaerobic bacteria and unusual organisms such as *Pasteurella multocida*, a human pathogen that is part of the normal oral flora of cats. Human bites are often associated with greater damage to the skin and soft tissues and are also polymicrobial with aerobic and anaerobic bacteria. Co-amoxiclav is an effective treatment for all these infections (Table 23.1).

Diabetic foot infections

Infections of the feet are particularly common in diabetics because several important host defences, including circulation and sensation, are compromised. This enables minor injuries to progress to advanced stages of infection rapidly and with very few symptoms. Consequently it is vital to educate patients with diabetes about how to avoid trauma to the feet and how to recognize infection early. Patients with diabetes also have impaired healing so that chronic ulcers are common.

Chronic ulcers without spreading cellulitis do not require antibiotic treatment, even if there is some purulence in the exudate as this simply indicates bacterial colonization of the ulcer. If there is cellulitis spreading up to 2 cm from the margin of the ulcer the infection is likely to respond to oral antibiotics, but if the infection spreads more widely or is associated with signs of sepsis then referral to hospital for intravenous treatment should be considered. Taking swabs from chronic ulcers is not helpful because they will be colonized with possibly harmless bacteria; even if infection is present the bacteria cultured are not always the ones that are responsible. Meaningful cultures can be obtained only by debriding the ulcer and then obtaining tissue specimens from the base of the lesion by curettage (scrapings with a sterile blade). Empirical treatment should cover both aerobic and anaerobic pathogens (Table 23.1).

Because of the combination of impaired circulation and sensation diabetic foot infections are particularly likely to progress to osteomyelitis because they may be present for weeks before the patient seeks medical attention. Osteomyelitis should be considered as a potential complication of any deep or extensive ulcer, especially if it is overlying a bony prominence or contains visible bone particles. Management of osteomyelitis is considered in Chapter 24.

Toxic shock syndrome

Certain phage types of *Staph. aureus* and *Str. pyogenes* produce toxins that cause a multisystem disease characterized by the sudden onset of fever, myalgia, vomiting, diarrhoea, hypotension, and an erythematous rash: the toxic shock syndrome. Staphylococcal toxic shock syndrome was originally thought to affect only menstruating women who used a particular type of tampon, it is now known to be a rare sequel of any type of staphylococcal infection. An antistaphylococcal penicillin (e.g. flucloxacillin) or clindamycin should be given, but antibiotic therapy is secondary to systemic support. Clinical results with intravenous immunoglobulin are inconsistent, probably because different batches of immunoglobulin contain variable quantities of neutralizing antibodies to some of these toxins.

Miscellaneous infections

Viral infections of the skin, such as herpes simplex and varicella zoster, are discussed in Chapter 27. Superficial fungal infections usually respond to topical therapy (Chapter 31), although dermatophyte infections of finger- or toenails may require oral treatment with terbinafine for up to 3 months, or with griseofulvin for a year or more. These agents are deposited in newly formed keratin and the prolonged treatment is needed to allow healthy nail to replace the diseased tissue. Even so, treatment of chronic infections of toenails may be unsuccessful, although terbinafine is more reliable in this respect than griseofulvin.

Further reading

Lipsky BA, Berendt AR, Deery HG, Embil JM, Joseph WS, Karchmer AW, LeFrock JL, Lew DP, Mader JT, Norden C, Tan JS. Diagnosis and treatment of diabetic foot infections. *Clinical Infectious Diseases* 2004; **39**:885–910.

Stevens DL, Bisno AL, Chambers HF, Everett ED, Dellinger P, Goldstein EJ, Gorbach SL, Hirschmann JV, Kaplan EL, Montoya JG, Wade JC. Practice guidelines for the diagnosis and management of skin and soft-tissue infections. *Clinical Infectious Diseases* 2005; **41**:1373–1406.

Chapter 24

Bone and joint infections

Septic arthritis

Bacteria can infect joints via the bloodstream (haematogenous septic arthritis) from a distant focus of infection such as a septic skin lesion, otitis media, pneumonia, meningitis, gonorrhoea, or an infection of the urinary tract. However, in adults prosthetic joint infection is now by far the most common presentation. Rarely bacteria may be introduced directly into the synovial space following a penetrating wound or an intra-articular injection. Also, the joint may become infected by direct spread from an adjacent area of osteomyelitis or cellulitis. Once established, septic arthritis can give rise to secondary bacteraemia.

Aetiology

Haematogenous septic arthritis

Staphylococcus aureus accounts for most bacteriologically proven joint infections. Other bacteria are important in specific age groups. *Escherichia coli* and streptococci of Lancefield group B (*Streptococcus agalactiae*) occur in neonates. Pneumococci, *Str. pyogenes*, and coliform bacilli are found in elderly people. *Haemophilus influenzae* of serotype b cause septicaemia and pyogenic arthritis in children under the age of 6 but childhood immunization with the *H. influenzae* conjugate vaccine has markedly reduced the incidence of this infection. *Neisseria gonorrhoeae* occasionally causes septic arthritis in young adults. Patients with meningococcal infection may develop septic arthritis during the course of their illness. Other rare causes include *Mycobacterium tuberculosis*, opportunist mycobacteria, *Brucella* spp., fungi, and *Borrelia burgdorferi*, the spirochaete that causes Lyme disease.

Prosthetic joint infection

Acute infections (within 1 year of the primary operation) are often caused by *Staph. aureus* or *Str. pyogenes*. Infections occurring more than a year after surgery are caused by a much wider range of bacteria, including coagulase negative staphylococci, enterococci, aerobic Gram-negative bacilli and anaerobic bacteria.

Management

Haematogenous septic arthritis

In nine cases out of 10 a single joint is involved, most commonly the knee, followed by the hip. Typically, the patient is a child with a high temperature and a red, hot, swollen joint with restricted movement. However, septic arthritis is not uncommon in elderly and debilitated people, who may have non-specific symptoms. Patients with rheumatoid arthritis have an increased incidence of septic arthritis and a poorer prognosis, which may in part be attributable to delay in making the clinical diagnosis.

A presumptive diagnosis rests on the immediate examination of the joint fluid, because of the difficulty on clinical grounds in distinguishing other conditions with similar features, such as an exacerbation of rheumatoid arthritis, gout, acute rheumatic fever, or trauma to the joint. Typically, the fluid is cloudy or purulent with a marked excess of neutrophils. The Gram film is of immediate help not only in confirming the diagnosis but also in the choice of the most appropriate antimicrobial therapy (Table 24.1). Despite the microscopic evidence of bacterial infection, culture of synovial fluid may sometimes fail to yield the pathogen, and blood cultures should always be taken at the same time. In suspected gonococcal arthritis, cervical, urethral, rectal, and throat swabs should also be taken for culture before starting antimicrobial therapy.

In young adults who present with acute mono-arthritis but do not have purulent joint fluid a diagnosis of reactive arthritis secondary to sexually transmitted disease should be suspected (Chapter 29).

It is very important that a diagnosis is made rapidly and appropriate therapy started immediately, because permanent damage to the joint may occur and lead to long-term residual abnormalities. Most patients who are treated promptly recover completely. Infection of the hip joint is more difficult to treat since, in addition to antibiotics, open surgical drainage is needed because of the technical difficulty of needle aspiration. The key to success is a combination of antibiotics and drainage. In most cases this is achieved by multidisciplinary management, including input from orthopaedic surgeons, medical microbiologists, and physicians. Surgeons in particular should determine whether drainage of pus should be by repeated needle aspiration or wash-out of the joint in an operating theatre.

The choice of initial antibiotic therapy depends on the age of the patient and the findings in the Gram-film. If organisms can be identified with reasonable confidence before culture, the appropriate antibiotic for that particular organism is the automatic choice irrespective of

Table 24.1 Initial antimicrobial therapy in septic arthritis when bacteria are seen in the Gram-film of the joint aspirate

Description of the Gram-film	Probable organism	Initial choice of antibiotic	Comments
Gram-positive cocci in clusters	Staphylococci	Flucloxacillin	Clindamycin if penicillin-allergic
Gram-positive cocci in chains or pairs	Streptococci	Benzylpenicillin	Clindamycin if penicillin-allergic
Gram-negative coccobacilli	H. influenzae	Fluoroquinolone	May change to ampicillin if sensitive
Gram-negative large rods	Coliform bacilli or Pseudomonas	Fluoroquinolone	Modify according to culture results
Gram-negative diplococci	Neisseria spp.	Benzylpenicillin	Ciprofloxacin if penicillin allergic or resistant

the age (Table 24.1). If bacteria are not seen at this stage, the initial choice is influenced by the age of the patient or the underlying disease. Antibiotics are chosen to cover the most likely bacterial causes of the infection (Table 24.2) and can be modified subsequently if a pathogen is isolated.

Most antimicrobial agents given parenterally achieve therapeutic levels in the infected joint, so the intra-articular injection of antibiotics is not recommended, particularly as it may induce chemical synovitis.

A sequential intravenous–oral regimen, carefully monitored at the time of oral therapy, is widely used. In all cases, the initial treatment must be with parenteral antibiotics until the condition of the patient has stabilized (usually 7–10 days) and the joint is reasonably dry. Switch to oral therapy is appropriate once the condition has stabilized as all of the first choice drugs are well absorbed after oral administration. The total duration of treatment is usually between 4 and 8 weeks and should be determined by clinicians who are experienced in management of these infections.

Prosthetic joint infection

Most patients with prosthetic joint infection are not systemically unwell. Infection should be suspected in any patient who develops pain or signs of local inflammation in the joint, although it is impossible to distinguish between mechanical loosening of the joint and infection unless there are obvious signs of infection such as purulent discharge from a sinus.

Table 24.2 Initial antimicrobial therapy in septic arthritis when no organisms are seen in the Gram-film of the joint aspirate

Type of patient	Most common organisms	Less common organisms	Initial choice of antibiotic
Neonate (0–2 months)	Staph. aureus Group B streptococci Gram-negative bacilli		Flucloxacillin[b] + gentamicin
Infant (2 months– 6 years)	Staph. aureus	Str. pyogenes Str. pneumoniae H. influenzae[a]	Flucloxacillin[b] + cefotaxime
Child (7–14 years)	Staph. aureus	MRSA	Flucloxacillin[b]
Adult (>15 years)	Staph. aureus	N. gonorrhoeae, MRSA	Flucloxacillin[b]
Elderly or debilitated	Staph. aureus	Str. pyogenes Str. pneumoniae MRSA Gram-negative bacilli	Flucloxacillin[b] + gentamicin

MRSA, methicillin-resistant Staph. aureus.

[a]Now rare where vaccine has been introduced.

[b]Vancomycin if MRSA likely.

Because there is rarely systemic illness it is not necessary to start empirical treatment and the chances of establishing a definitive microbiological diagnosis are greatly enhanced if antibiotics are not given. Serious systemic illness is the only reason for giving empirical antibiotics, as it is extremely unlikely that prosthetic joint infection will resolve with antibiotic therapy alone.

Patients with suspected prosthetic joint infection should be referred urgently to an orthopaedic surgeon who specializes in revision surgery for prosthetic joints and who is likely to work closely with medical microbiologists and infectious diseases physicians.

Osteomyelitis

Osteomyelitis is infection of bone and is usually caused by bacteria. Unlike soft tissues, bone is a rigid structure and cannot swell. As infection proceeds and pus forms, there is a marked rise of pressure in the affected part of the bone, which, if unchecked or unrelieved, may impair the blood supply to a wide area and result in areas of infected dead bone. Once this chronic phase of osteomyelitis is established, necrotic bone (sequestrum) must be removed surgically in addition to the use of antibiotics if the infection is to be eradicated.

Pathogenesis and aetiology

Osteomyelitis may be haematogenous (infected through the bloodstream) or non-haematogenous (infected directly through a wound, including a fracture or an overlying chronic ulcer).

Haematogenous osteomyelitis

This type of infection is most commonly caused by staphylococci that reach the site through the bloodstream, usually with no obvious primary focus of infection. Acute haematogenous osteomyelitis is principally a disease of children under 16 years, in whom more than 85% of cases occur. The usual sites are the long bones (femur, tibia, humerus) near the metaphysis, where the blood supply to the bone is most dense. However, when the disease occurs in adults, the vertebrae are commonly affected.

Staph. aureus accounts for about half of all cases and for more than 90% of cases in otherwise normal children. In the elderly with underlying malignancies and other diseases, and in drug addicts, Gram-negative bacilli (coliform bacilli and *Ps. aeruginosa*) are reported with increasing frequency. Coliforms are particularly likely to cause vertebral osteomyelitis, as it is associated with recurrent urinary tract infection. *H. influenzae* has become very rare since the introduction of the conjugate vaccine. Other rare causes of haematogenous osteomyelitis include *M. tuberculosis*, *Brucella abortus*, and, particularly in parts of the world where sickle-cell anaemia is prevalent, salmonellae.

Non-haematogenous osteomyelitis

When bones are infected by the introduction of organisms through traumatic or postoperative wounds, *Staph. aureus* is still the commonest cause, but Gram-negative bacteria may also be found. *Ps. aeruginosa* may occasionally produce osteomyelitis of the metatarsals or calcaneum following a puncture wound of the sole of the foot and *Pasteurella multocida* infection may follow animal bites. Patients with infected pressure sores over a bone, or those with peripheral vascular disease or diabetes mellitus, may develop osteomyelitis with mixed aerobic and anaerobic organisms (coliforms and *Bacteroides* species), although *Staph. aureus* is an important cause of osteomyelitis by this route also.

Clinical and diagnostic considerations

The typical manifestations of acute, haematogenous osteomyelitis include the abrupt onset of high fever and systemic toxicity, with marked redness, pain, and swelling over the bone involved. In vertebral osteomyelitis, there may be general malaise, with or without low-grade fever and low back pain. If the infection is not controlled, it may spread to produce a spinal epidural abscess, with consequent neurological symptoms.

The diagnosis of osteomyelitis is confirmed by bone biopsy. A bone scan may help to localize the site and extent of the infection. However, bone scan is simply a demonstration of increased blood supply to the affected area and cannot distinguish between infection and other causes of inflammation. A positive bone scan should be a stimulus to further investigation, whereas a negative bone scan makes the diagnosis of osteomyelitis unlikely. Magnetic resonance imaging provides additional information about the presence and location of a sequestrum. Blood cultures should be taken in addition to bone biopsy. In patients with chronic osteomyelitis, it may be misleading to base antibiotic treatment on the results of cultures of pus obtained from a draining sinus, which will often yield organisms that are secondarily colonizing the sinus. For precise bacteriological diagnosis, material must be obtained during the surgical removal of dead bone and tissue.

Guidelines for antibiotic therapy and management

It is generally agreed that acute haematogenous osteomyelitis can be cured without surgical intervention, provided antibiotics are given while the bone retains its blood supply and before extensive necrosis has occurred. In practice, this is within the first 72 h of the development of symptoms. Antibiotic therapy must, therefore, start immediately after a bone biopsy and blood cultures have been obtained. Results from a Gram-film of aspirated material may help in the initial choice of antibiotic. If no organisms are seen *Staph. aureus* is the prime suspect in any age group, and an antistaphylococcal agent should be used (flucloxacillin or clindamycin). If Gram-negative bacteria are isolated a fluoroquinolone is the drug of choice.

To ensure adequate concentration at the site of infection, high doses of antibiotics should be given parenterally. If an abscess has already formed when the patient is first seen, or there is no significant clinical improvement within 24 h of starting parenteral therapy, then surgical drainage of the abscess is essential.

The details of treatment, including duration of intravenous therapy and total duration of treatment should be determined by specialists with experience in the management of these complex conditions.

Chapter 25

Mycobacterial disease

Tuberculosis

Tuberculosis (TB) is one of the most widespread human infections. The World Health Organization (WHO) estimate that a third of the world's population harbour *Mycobacterium tuberculosis*, and every year more than eight million people develop new clinical disease. The pulmonary form was described by Hippocrates, and characteristic lesions of TB of the spine have been demonstrated in the mummies of ancient Egypt. The disease attacks both man and animals, affects all ages and every organ in the body, and ranges from latent to hyperacute (the 'galloping consumption' of Victorian times), killing young and old alike, the famous and the unknown. This reservoir of infected persons is made up of those with infectious pulmonary TB (sputum-smear positive) who can infect between 10 and 15 people every year. Co-infection with human immunodeficiency virus (HIV) is the most potent risk factor for the development of active TB: according to the WHO over 40 million people are co-infected.

The last 60 years have seen enormous progress in the understanding of the epidemiology, prevention, and treatment of TB and, although far from eradicated, this age-old killer of man has become a preventable and curable disease. The prevalence in a population is linked to a number of socio-economic factors, notably poverty, malnutrition, social exclusion, and poor health services. Furthermore, the HIV pandemic has magnified the impact of TB, particularly in sub-Saharan Africa, where co-infection rates are greatest. The control of TB is a global healthcare priority and cannot be successful unless HIV prevention and control become parallel priorities.

Immune response

Immunity in TB is cell mediated; the key to restriction of intracellular growth of the bacillus is co-operation between macrophages and sensitized lymphocytes. Humoral reactions are thought to play little part. The generation of clones of antigen-specific T cells initiates the immune response, which is depressed in HIV-positive patients. T-cell clones may facilitate elimination of the pathogen by macrophage activation and granuloma formation or by cytotoxic action; or they may interact with B cells to produce specific antibodies, which, in conjunction with phagocytic cells or complement, also act as an effector arm. The mechanism by which mycobacteria survive inside activated macrophages is unknown and may be oxygen dependent or oxygen independent. A genetic predisposition to tuberculous disease has been sought. Certain HLA-haplotypes have been associated with heightened susceptibility.

Principles of management

TB can affect many organs and tissues (Table 25.1). However, the pulmonary form of the disease is most common (65%) and accounts for its spread. The effective management of pulmonary TB therefore remains the greatest priority in controlling this disease. The key components of management are:

- rapid detection of active disease;
- reliable microbiological diagnosis;
- supervised treatment with combination chemotherapy;
- notification of cases and contact tracing;
- monitoring for drug-resistant disease;
- continuous reporting and surveillance.

Vaccination is included in this strategy by some countries, including the UK. The vaccine is based on a laboratory-modified strain of *M. bovis*, which is administered as BCG (bacille Calmette–Guérin—named after the two French originators of the vaccine). However, the efficacy of this vaccine has proved highly variable in published studies. Furthermore, it requires pre-immunization Mantoux test screening of the recipients using tuberculin (an extract of *M. tuberculosis*) to distinguish between previously infected (positive tuberculin test) and non-infected (negative tuberculin test) persons. Because of the logistics of testing, and the occasional difficulty in interpreting the skin test outcome, together with the fact that the vaccine sensitizes recipients to tuberculin thus reducing its value in skin testing to identify

Table 25.1 Tuberculosis: presenting infections

Common	Less common	Uncommon
Pulmonary	Meningitis	Pericardial
Lymph node	Intra-abdominal	Skin
Genito-urinary	Bone	

at-risk persons, many countries have not adopted this approach. In the UK BCG immunization is now restricted to babies and older people who are most at risk of TB, such as those living in areas with a high rate of TB or whose parents or grandparents were born in countries with a high prevalence of the disease.

Clinical diagnosis

Symptoms of persistent cough, often with minimal sputum production, occasional coughing up of blood (haemoptysis), weight loss, and sweats (often at night) should all raise suspicions for pulmonary TB. A chest X-ray will often show evidence of diffuse upper lobe streaking and consolidation. More advanced disease results in cavity formation.

Microbiological diagnosis

Specimens, notably sputum from patients with suspected pulmonary TB, should be examined microscopically using either a fluorescent stain (auramine) or the more traditional Ziehl–Neelsen stain. The microscopic detection of bacilli with the typical appearances of *M. tuberculosis* permits early diagnosis. Such a patient is classified as 'smear-positive' and managed as if they have 'open' (contagious) TB.

Other samples for diagnosis include biopsy material (lymph node, bone marrow, other tissues). Culture of *M. tuberculosis* is slow and may take 3–6 weeks to confirm the diagnosis. Susceptibility testing of anti-TB drugs adds to the length of this process. Rapid methods of identification are becoming more widely available, including rapid tests of susceptibility to isoniazid and rifampicin.

Treatment

The chemotherapy of human TB has depended almost entirely on large prospective controlled trials of different regimens, which have helped define the current recommendations for the treatment and prevention of the disease. There is still no in-vitro or animal model that can reliably predict the response to treatment in man.

Standard first-line treatment for TB requires compliance with a multidrug regimen for a minimum period of 6 months. Rifampicin and isoniazid are potent anti-TB agents and are administered throughout the 6 months. Pyrazinamide is added for the initial 2 months. A further drug, such as ethambutol is also included for the first 2 months if there are concerns about drug-resistant disease, with streptomycin as a further alternative (Table 25.2).

The rationale for this multidrug regimen is to provide effective therapy while avoiding the emergence of naturally occurring low frequency drug-resistant mutant strains of *M. tuberculosis*, which may cause relapse of the disease following the eradication of the susceptible strains. The initial 3–4 drug regimen is effective in preventing this from happening. Under normal circumstances, culture and sensitivity information should be available by 2 months to permit the safe transfer to rifampicin and isoniazid for the final 4 months of treatment.

Multidrug-resistant TB, defined as resistance to both isoniazid and rifampicin, is increasing worldwide. It currently accounts for less than 5% of isolates in the UK but has reached very high levels (> 35%) in parts of Russia and some eastern European countries. This is of major concern since laboratory facilities to support the clinical management of TB in resource poor countries are often inadequate and coincide with highest incidence rates of disease, including that caused by multiresistant TB. Second-line agents for treating TB (Table 25.3) are not only less active but often more toxic than first-line drugs. Treatment must also be prolonged for periods of up to 18–24 months.

Treatment of TB requires close supervision and should be under the direction of a specialist in respiratory medicine or infectious diseases and

Table 25.2 Recommended first line treatment regimens for tuberculosis in adults

Drug	Initial phase (2 months)	Continuation phase (4 months)	Major side effects
Standard regimen			
Rifampicin	10 mg/kg/day (450–600 mg/day)	10 mg/kg/day (450–600 mg/day)	Hepatitis; gastrointestinal upsets
Isoniazid[a]	5 mg/kg/day (200–300 mg/day)	5 mg/kg/day (200–300 mg/day)	Peripheral neuropathy; hepatitis
Pyrazinamide	30 mg/kg/day (1.5–2 g/day)		Gastrointestinal upsets; gout
Ethambutol	15–25 mg/kg/day		Retrobulbar neuritis
Intermittent regimen (3 times weekly)			
Rifampicin	10 mg/kg	10 mg/kg	As above
Isoniazid	15 mg/kg	15 mg/kg	
Pyrazinamide	50 mg/kg	50 mg/kg	

[a]Or streptomycin (15 mg/kg/day or 0.75–1 g/day for 2 months if resistant to isoniazid).

intramuscular injection. It is more bactericidal during the proliferative phase than in the resting phase of bacterial growth. Adequate concentrations are attained in lung, muscle, uterus, intestinal mucosa, adrenals, and lymph nodes. Diffusion into bone, brain, and aqueous humour is poor. Little normally enters the CSF, although penetration increases when the meninges are inflamed. The deep intramuscular injections are painful and must be administered daily for up to 2 months.

Ototoxicity is the most serious adverse reaction. Vestibular damage occurs in about 30% of cases while cochleotoxicity is less common. The plasma half-life is normally 2–3 h, but is considerably extended in the newborn, in the elderly, and in patients with severe renal impairment. Serum levels need to be monitored in patients over 40 years of age. The dose is adjusted for age and renal function. Hypersensitivity reactions in the form of fever and skin rashes may develop.

Second-line drugs

Thiacetazone

Thiacetazone is one of the earliest anti-TB drugs, and is cheap to manufacture. It is bacteristatic against *M. tuberculosis* and is sometimes used in combination with isoniazid to inhibit the emergence of resistance, particularly in the continuation phase of long-term regimens. It is well absorbed from the gastrointestinal tract and plasma levels are sustained for long periods of time. Side effects include nausea, vomiting, diarrhoea, skin rashes, and bone marrow depression. Rare cases of fatal exfoliative dermatitis and acute hepatitis failure have been reported.

Ethionamide and protionamide

Because of its gastrointestinal side effects—anorexia, salivation, nausea, abdominal pain, and diarrhoea—ethionamide is one of the most unpleasant of all anti-TB drugs to take and is no longer recommended. Protionamide is closely related in structure, and is better tolerated. It is absorbed quickly when given by mouth with good tissue and CSF levels. It is bacteristatic at therapeutic concentrations but bactericidal at higher concentrations. Contra-indications include pregnancy, severe liver damage, and gastric complaints; care should be exercised in epilepsy and in psychotic patients. Combinations with isoniazid, cycloserine, or alcohol should be avoided.

Cycloserine, amikacin, kanamycin, and capreomycin

These are four rather weak drugs used as reserves for the treatment of TB resistant to the first-line agents. Capreomycin, amikacin, and kanamycin all need to be given by injection. Primary resistance is rare but resistance can develop rapidly.

Fluoroquinolones

Several fluoroquinolones are active against *M. tuberculosis*. They include ciprofloxacin, ofloxacin, levofloxacin and moxifloxacin. They are bactericidal, orally administered, and well tolerated. They are increasingly being used in the treatment of drug-resistant TB.

p-Aminosalicylic acid

This was formerly used in combination regimens to prevent the emergence of drug-resistant organisms. Up to 10–12 g a day were given orally, in two or three doses. The drug tastes most unpleasant, and gastrointestinal intolerance was common. *p*-Aminosalicylic acid is no longer used and is included here for historical reasons only.

Short course and intermittent therapy

The discovery that both pyrazinamide and rifampicin are active against dormant as well as actively dividing tubercle bacilli prompted the investigation of shorter periods of treatment. Based on clinical trials, it has been shown that all regimens containing two of the three drugs, isoniazid, pyrazinamide, and rifampicin cure more than 90% of patients in 6 months and virtually all in 9 months. The limitations of treatment are those of cost and of patient compliance. In developing countries, short course intermittent therapy permits supervised mass treatment at a cost the communities can afford.

Affluent countries have slightly different aims. These countries require highly effective unsupervised regimens for use where patient motivation is high and compliance good. The standard regimen of treatment recommended by the British Thoracic Society is an initial phase of 2 months treatment with rifampicin, isoniazid, plus pyrazinamide and ethambutol, then a continuation phase of treatment with isoniazid and rifampicin for a further 4 months (Table 25.2). The regimen of three or four drugs during the initial intensive phase of treatment is important in bringing the acute illness under control as rapidly as possible.

Intermittent regimens have become popular in developing countries for ease of administration. Rifampicin in standard dose, together with isoniazid and pyrazinamide at doses higher than the standard regimen are given on 3 days of the week, again for a total of 6 months (Table 25.2).

maculopapular. Blood cultures are positive in about 40% of cases. With appropriate treatment, mortality is 3–5%.

Rarer forms of meningococcal disease

Occasionally *N. meningitidis* may localize in the joints or on heart valves producing acute septic arthritis or endocarditis. Chronic meningococcal septicaemia, although uncommon, is characterized by intermittent pyrexia, rash, and arthralgia. Occasionally a diagnosis is made retrospectively because of transient positive blood cultures in children with mild, self-limiting, febrile illness. They usually recover quickly and spontaneously without the use of antibiotics.

Treatment and prophylaxis

Ceftriaxone is the drug of choice. Therapy should be started on first suspicion of meningococcal disease. Although most strains of *N. meningitidis* are highly sensitive to penicillin (minimum inhibitory concentration <0.16 mg/l), some strains of reduced sensitivity are occasionally encountered and hence the reason why ceftriaxone is the preferred agent.

To prevent secondary cases of meningococcal disease, household and secretion (kissing) contacts are offered antibiotic prophylaxis. The standard agent for prophylaxis is oral rifampicin, twice daily for 2 days (adults 600 mg; children 10 mg/kg). Rifampicin-resistant strains occur, but are presently uncommon. A single intramuscular injection of ceftriaxone (adults 250 mg; children 125 mg) or a single oral dose of ciprofloxacin (adults 500 mg) are alternative prophylactic regimens. Pregnant women should be offered ceftriaxone rather than rifampicin.

Pneumococcal meningitis

Meningitis caused by *Str. pneumoniae* may occur at any age. The mortality in children and adults is about 20 and 35% respectively. The outlook is grave in those over the age of 60 years. There is often a pre-existing focus of infection elsewhere (e.g. pneumonia, acute otitis media, or acute sinusitis), predisposing risk factor (e.g. recent or remote head trauma, recent neuro-surgical procedure, CSF leak, sickle cell anaemia, an immunodeficiency state, alcoholism, or an absent spleen). *Str. pneumoniae* is the commonest cause of recurrent or post-traumatic meningitis. Patients who have had a splenectomy are at particular risk of developing overwhelming pneumococcal infection. The onset of pneumococcal meningitis may be sudden and the course rapid with death occurring within 12 h. Alterations of consciousness and focal neurological defects may occur and survivors often suffer significant neurological deficits.

Treatment

Ceftriaxone is the preferred agent to treat pneumococcal meningitis. The increasing worldwide incidence of penicillin-resistant pneumococci has eroded the efficacy of benzylpenicillin, which was formerly the drug of choice. Strains of pneumococci that are resistant to expanded-spectrum cephalosporins such as ceftriaxone are being increasingly reported from around the world but are currently rare in the UK; rifampicin or vancomycin have been used in such cases, but are less than ideal.

The duration of treatment is at least 10 days, but is extended up to 14 days in young infants or in complicated cases.

Haemophilus meningitis

Almost all cases of meningitis due to *H. influenzae* are caused by the capsulate type b strains. Before the introduction of the highly successful conjugate vaccine, *H. influenzae* meningitis affected children under 6 years of age, reflecting the absence of anticapsular antibody in this age group. The mortality was about 7%. The onset of *H. influenzae* meningitis is often insidious, progressing over a period of 3–5 days. In some infants the illness may be limited to fever, vomiting, and diarrhoea in the early stages, making diagnosis of meningitis difficult.

Treatment and prophylaxis

Cefotaxime or ceftriaxone, which are active against β-lactamase-producing and non-β-lactamase-producing strains of *H. influenzae* are the agents of choice for treatment. Rifampicin is used as prophylaxis for all household contacts when there is an unvaccinated sibling in the house aged 4 years or younger.

Neonatal meningitis

The highest risk of developing meningitis in the newborn is within the first 2 months of life, the incidence being about 0.3 per 1000 live births. Neonatal meningitis carries a high mortality. The incidence of neurological deficits in those who survive is also depressingly high. Brain abscess is a rare complication.

Predisposing factors include prematurity, low birth weight, prolonged and difficult labour, prolonged rupture of membranes, and maternal perinatal infection. Some cases complicate congenital defects of the neuraxis.

Neonatal meningitis is usually the result of vertical transfer of pathogens from the mother in utero or during delivery, leading to early-onset (occurring within 7 days of delivery) septicaemia or meningitis; less commonly they are acquired from the environment, leading to late-onset meningitis (occurring after 7 days and occasionally up to 2 months after delivery). Early-onset disease often presents as an overwhelming septicaemia with apnoea and shock. The pulmonary manifestations may be difficult to differentiate from respiratory distress syndrome. Meningitis occurs in 30% of cases. About 1 in 100 newborns colonized with group B streptococci develop early-onset disease; mortality is over 50%. Late-onset disease usually presents as meningitis and mortality is about 20%.

The early signs and symptoms are often non-specific and include fever, lethargy, and refusal of feed. A bulging fontanelle, resulting from raised intracranial pressure, is a relatively late sign. A high degree of suspicion and prompt investigation with lumbar puncture is essential. Of those who survive, about half will have evidence of neurological damage.

Treatment

Neonatal meningitis is more difficult to treat, since a wide variety of organisms may be involved and their susceptibility to antibiotics can be unpredictable. The chosen therapy should be supported by appropriate laboratory tests.

Group B haemolytic streptococci

The treatment of choice is high dose benzylpenicillin for at least 2 weeks. Some strains show enhanced killing in vitro when benzylpenicillin is combined with gentamicin, which may be given for the first 7–10 days.

Escherichia coli and other enterobacteria

The most widely used regimen is high-dose cefotaxime in combination with gentamicin to provide synergistic bactericidal activity against *Esch. coli* or other enterobacteria. Ceftriaxone together with gentamicin is preferred for meningitis caused by salmonellae, and ceftazidime plus gentamicin for *Pseudomonas aeruginosa*. The duration of treatment should be at least 3 weeks.

Listeria monocytogenes

This is a Gram-positive bacillus that exists as a soil saprophyte in nature. Infection is probably acquired from dairy or vegetable produce contaminated from animal sources. The organism may be carried asymptomatically in the gastrointestinal or the female genital tract. The neonate may be infected transplacentally in utero or from the genital tract during delivery. Bacteraemia may occur in a pregnant woman following a flu-like illness, which might result in intrauterine infection of the fetus leading to abortion and stillbirth, or the baby may develop symptoms of disseminated infection a few days after delivery. Neonatal mortality with intrauterine listeriosis is about 30%. Most cases of late-onset infection present as meningitis in a previously normal neonate.

L. monocytogenes also causes meningitis in adults, particularly in the elderly, the immunocompromised, or those with an underlying disease. Occasionally the disease occurs in previously healthy adults of all ages.

The organism is sensitive to a variety of agents, but the treatment of choice is high-dose ampicillin with or without gentamicin. In adults with a history of penicillin allergy, intravenous or oral co-trimoxazole (which is bactericidal to *L. monocytogenes*) should be substituted, with chloramphenicol as a further alternative. Cephalosporins have no useful activity against *L. monocytogenes*.

The duration of therapy should be 3 weeks since cerebritis may accompany the meningitis and requires more prolonged treatment.

A summary of current recommendations for the initial therapy of the commoner forms of bacterial meningitis is outlined in Table 26.4.

Viral and parasitic encephalitis

The treatment of herpes simplex encephalitis and African trypanosomiasis are discussed in Chapters 27 and 30 respectively.

Rarer forms of meningitis

Staphylococcus aureus

Meningitis due to *Staph. aureus* may occur in patients with fulminating septicaemia secondary to pneumonia or endocarditis, or as a complication of penetrating head injury, recent neurosurgical procedures (including insertion of shunts), and ruptured cerebral or epidural abscess. Mortality is high and neurological sequelae are common in survivors.

Most *Staph. aureus* strains are resistant to penicillin. For methicillin-sensitive strains high-dose flucloxacillin (at least 12 g daily) combined with oral rifampicin (600 mg daily) is recommended in adults. In patients who are allergic to penicillin or in meningitis due to methicillin-resistant strains, treatment is even more problematic. Parenteral vancomycin (1 g every 12 h) combined with oral rifampicin is recommended. However, since penetration of vancomycin into the CSF is limited, daily intraventricular vancomycin should also be considered. Intraventricular vancomycin is also warranted in meningitis with methicillin-sensitive strains if the CSF is persistently positive despite flucloxacillin and rifampicin, and in patients with shunt-associated meningitis. The duration of treatment for *Staph aureus* meningitis should be at least 3 weeks.

Table 26.4 Antibiotic treatment of the common types of bacterial meningitis

Age	Cerebrospinal fluid Gram-film findings	Presumptive organism	Treatment of choice			Comments
			Antibiotic(s)	Daily dose (interval)	Duration	
<2 months	Gram-positive cocci in chains	Group B streptococci	Benzylpenicillin + gentamicin[a]	200 mg/kg (6 h)	2 weeks	In selected patients, gentamicin may be discontinued after 7–10 days
	Gram-negative bacilli	'Coliforms' (usually Esch. coli)	Cefotaxime + gentamicin[a]	200 mg/kg (6 h)	3 weeks	Change to ceftriaxone if Salmonella, or ceftazidime if Ps. aeruginosa
	Gram-positive bacilli	L. monocytogenes	Ampicillin + gentamicin[a]	200 mg/kg (6 h)	3 weeks	Rare cause of neonatal meningitis
	No organisms seen	Any of the above	Cefotaxime ± gentamicin[a] ± ampicillin	200 mg/kg (6 h) 200 mg/kg (6 h)	Variable[b]	Ampicillin added if L. monocytogenes strongly suspected

(continued)

TABLE 26.4 (continued) Antibiotic treatment of the common types of bacterial meningitis

Age	Cerebrospinal fluid Gram-film findings	Presumptive organism	Treatment of choice		Duration	Comments
			Antibiotic(s)	Daily dose (interval)		
2 months–6 years	Gram-negative diplococci	N. meningitidis	Benzylpenicillin	300 mg/kg (4 h)	7 days	Cefotaxime if allergic to penicillin
	Gram-positive diplococci	Str. pneumoniae	Benzylpenicillin	300 mg/kg (4 h)	10 days	Cefotaxime or ceftriaxone if allergic to penicillin[c]; in young infants and complicated cases treatment may be extended up to 2 weeks
	Gram-negative coccobacilli	H. influenzae	Cefotaxime or ceftriaxone	200 mg/kg (6 h) / 80 mg/kg (24 h)	10 days	Chloramphenicol in patients with severe cephalosporin allergy
	No organisms seen	Any of the above 3	Cefotaxime or ceftriaxone	200 mg/kg (6 h) / 80 mg/kg (24 h)	Variable[b]	Change as appropriate according to culture result
>6–40 years	Gram-negative diplococci	N. meningitidis	Benzylpenicillin	Child: as above Adult: 14.4 g (4 h)	7 days	As above
	Gram-positive diplococci	Str. pneumoniae	Benzylpenicillin	As above	10 days	As above[c]
	No organisms seen	Either of the above 2	Ceftriaxone	80 mg/kg (24 h)	Variable[b]	

Age	Gram stain	Organism	Antibiotic	Dose	Duration	Notes
>40 years	Gram-positive diplococci	Str. pneumoniae	Benzylpenicillin	14.4 g (4 h)	10 days	As above
	Gram-positive bacilli	L. monocytogenes	Ampicillin + gentamicin	12 g (4 h)	2–3 weeks	Co-trimoxazole if the patient allergic to penicillin
	Gram-negative bacilli	Esch. coli, etc	Cefotaxime + gentamicin	12 g (4 h)	3 weeks	Or ceftriaxone (4 g once daily) + gentamicin
	No organisms seen	Pneumococci or listeria	Ampicillin	12 g (4 h)	Variable[b]	Add flucloxacillin for neurosurgical patients; change as appropriate according to culture result
Any age	Gram-positive cocci in clusters	Staphylococci (usually Staph. aureus)	Flucloxacillin +	Adult: 12 g (4 h) Child: 200 mg/kg (4–6 h)	3–4 weeks	If shunt-associated removal of shunt usually necessary; vancomycin instead of flucloxacillin if: −patient penicillin allergic −MRSA −Staph. epidermidis isolated
			Rifampicin (oral)	Adult: 600 mg (12 h) Child: 20 mg/kg (12 h)		

MRSA, methicillin resistant Staph. aureus.

[a]In neonates with normal renal function, the unit dose is based on the body weight (usually 2.5 mg/kg) but the interval between the doses varies with the gestational age and the postnatal age (gestational age <28 weeks, 24h; 29–35 weeks, 18 h; 36–40 weeks, 12 h; >41 weeks, 8 h).

[b]Duration will depend on the organism isolated.

[c]Use cefotaxime or ceftriaxone also in areas of high prevalence of pneumococci with reduced susceptibility to penicillin.

Shunt-associated meningitis

In patients with hydrocephalus the ventricular CSF is diverted to other compartments of the body (usually the peritoneal cavity) with a silastic catheter (shunt). Unfortunately, 15–25% of these patients develop meningitis at some point in the life of the shunt. *Staph. epidermidis* accounts for about half and *Staph. aureus* for about a quarter of shunt infections. Among many other micro-organisms associated with such infections are *Propionibacterium acnes*, diphtheroids, enterococci, and Gram-negative bacilli. Most infections are believed to be due to colonization of the shunt at the time of surgery; occasionally organisms may reach the CSF and shunt through the bloodstream or by retrograde spread. Examination of the CSF obtained by needle aspiration of the reservoir is essential and yields an organism in over 90% of cases. It is not unusual to isolate bacteria from an otherwise normal CSF. Blood cultures are positive only if meningitis is associated with a ventriculo-atrial shunt.

Some patients who develop meningitis due to *N. meningitidis*, *H. influenzae*, or *Str. pneumoniae* are treated with appropriate antibiotics, without shunt removal. However, many infections will fail to be controlled unless there is complete removal of the shunt.

Since *Staph. epidermidis* is commonly resistant to flucloxacillin, therapy should be commenced with parenteral vancomycin combined with oral rifampicin and daily intraventricular vancomycin. High-dose flucloxacillin should be substituted for parenteral vancomycin if the isolate proves sensitive. Treatment should be continued for 2–3 weeks before a new shunt is inserted.

Mycobacterium tuberculosis

Tuberculous meningitis can affect any age. It is uncommon in developed countries and cases can be missed unless the physician is aware of the possibility and the laboratory is willing to exclude tuberculous meningitis in all cases in which abnormal clinical or CSF findings (increased lymphocytes, raised protein, low CSF glucose) have not been satisfactorily explained. The treatment of tuberculous meningitis is described in Chapter 25.

Cryptococcal meningitis

Cryptococcus neoformans is a saprophytic encapsulated fungus commonly found in soil and pigeon droppings. It is an uncommon cause of meningitis, occurring mainly in patients who are immunocompromised due to disease or drugs. Cryptococcal meningitis is reported to occur in about 4% of AIDS patients in the UK and up to a third of African patients with AIDS. It is probably transmitted via the respiratory tract. Most patients present with features of a subacute meningitis or meningo-encephalitis.

The treatment of cryptococcal CNS disease consists of an initial 2-week induction phase with intravenous amphotericin B, with or without flucytosine (by mouth or intravenously). Flucytosine is associated with more rapid sterilization of the CSF and fewer failures or relapses. Following induction, a consolidation phase with fluconazole is adopted. Alternative agents include amphotericin B or itraconazole. The total duration of treatment is determined by clinical response, monitoring levels of cryptococcal antigen in the blood and CSF and central nervous system imaging where appropriate. In those with underlying HIV infection and low CD4 counts fluconazole is used long term as chemoprophylaxis to prevent recurrent infection.

Culture-negative pyogenic meningitis

About 40% of patients presenting with meningitis will already have received antimicrobial therapy before lumbar puncture and this may lead to failure to isolate the organism. Prior therapy does not seriously alter cell counts or protein and glucose concentrations and it is usually still possible to differentiate between bacterial and viral meningitis. In about 10% of cases the aetiology remains unknown.

Although prior therapy may confuse the clinical picture it is not detrimental to the individual patient who has as good a prognosis as those who are untreated. 'Best guess' therapy should be aimed at common bacterial pathogens; ceftriaxone (or cefotaxime) for 7–14 days is a reasonable choice. The duration of therapy should be determined by clinical response and repeat CSF examination where appropriate. In the presence of an obvious meningococcal rash 7 days treatment is sufficient.

All patients in whom there is no history of previous antibiotic to account for the negative results must be investigated further to exclude conditions such as tuberculous or cryptococcal meningitis, superficial brain abscess, or other parameningeal infections.

Brain abscess

Brain abscess is a localized collection of pus within the brain parenchyma. It is a life-threatening condition, although the mortality has been reduced to less than 10% by the introduction of CT and magnetic resonance imaging, leading to earlier diagnosis and more precise localization; by improvements in surgical and bacteriological techniques; and by the use of appropriate antibiotics. About four to 10 cases a year are seen in neurological units of developed countries. Brain abscess in children accounts for less than 25% of all cases and, except in neonates, it is rare in those under 2 years of age.

Pathogenesis

Brain abscesses develop most commonly by spread of infection from an adjacent cranial site (e.g. paranasal sinuses, middle ear, mastoid, or teeth), following a penetrating cranial trauma or neurosurgery, or by haematogenous spread from a distant site (e.g. lung abscess, bronchiectasis, or endocarditis). Blood-borne spread often leads to multiple abscess formation. In about 20% of cases the primary focus of infection remains unrecognized—so-called cryptogenic abscess.

The organisms isolated usually reflect those found in the primary focus of infection. With proper attention to microbiological culture techniques, the role of anaerobes and polymicrobial infection has become apparent. Brain abscess in association with sinusitis is usually located in the frontal lobe and is most commonly caused by *Str. milleri* with or without anaerobes. In contrast, brain abscess following chronic suppurative otitis media or mastoiditis is usually located in the temporal lobe or cerebellum. The infection is invariably polymicrobial, and the pus obtained may yield a variety of anaerobic and aerobic bacteria. *Staph. aureus* is usually isolated in pure culture from brain abscess that has followed trauma or neurosurgery, or is secondary to a haematogenous spread from infective endocarditis, whereas *Str. milleri* together with anaerobes and other respiratory pathogens should be suspected in brain abscess complicating pyogenic lung abscess. Rare causes include *M. tuberculosis, L. monocytogenes, Nocardia asteroides, Toxoplasma gondii, Cryptococcus neoformans*, and other fungi.

Treatment

Although some patients with early cerebritis, or small, deep, or multiple abscesses have been treated successfully with antimicrobial therapy alone, most require surgical drainage. CT-guided stereotaxic aspiration allows more accurate drainage with minimal interference to the surrounding normal brain. Lumbar puncture is unhelpful in diagnosis and may be hazardous. Blood cultures may be positive and should be taken.

Pus obtained after any of these procedures requires prompt microscopy and culture. Because mixtures of aerobic and anaerobic bacteria are likely, antimicrobial therapy should cover both possibilities. Cefotaxime or other similar agents (ceftriaxone, ceftazidime) are recommended. When used in high doses these antibiotics penetrate well into brain abscess pus, and they are bactericidal against many of the organisms commonly encountered,

have a milder, shorter-lasting infection. About 70% of contacts given the drug are protected from infection. However, amantadine is unpopular in the elderly, who suffer the brunt of serious influenza, because of its stimulatory actions on the central nervous system. Patients become confused and agitated, and may be unable to sleep.

Amantadine may be of more use in the prevention of spread of infection in an institution in which influenza has already occurred. Vaccination of non-infected individuals may take 2 weeks to induce protection, whereas protection with amantadine is demonstrable after a few hours. The drug is also an alternative for those in whom vaccination is contra-indicated because of egg allergy or for other reasons.

Rimantadine, a derivative of amantadine, is said to be equipotent in its anti-influenzal properties but less prone to side effects. However, it is not currently licensed in the UK. Viral resistance emerges rapidly in patients treated with either of these drugs.

Influenza A and B viruses are sensitive to the neuraminidase inhibitors, zanamivir and oseltamivir, which are the preferred drugs to manage influenza virus infection. Controlled trials have shown a shorter time to the resolution of symptoms and lower usage of antibiotics among patients treated with these drugs. However, they must be given within 48 h of onset of symptoms for maximum benefit—a time frame not often met by patients suffering influenzal symptoms. Moreover, zanamivir has poor oral bioavailability, is not licensed for children under 12 years of age and has to be given by oral or nasal inhalation. Oseltamivir, in contrast, can be administered by mouth in capsules and a 5-day course is recommended. Currently in the UK, it is recommended that neuraminidase inhibitors be used when influenza is circulating in the community for 'at-risk' persons, which includes those with chronic respiratory, renal or cardiovascular disease, and diabetes mellitus together with the immunocompromised and those age 65 years or older.

Oseltamivir may also be prescribed prophylactically to prevent influenza in 'at-risk' children aged 1 year or older with similar criteria as above, provided prophylaxis can be started within 48 h of exposure. This is only practically possible when influenza virus is known to be circulating in the community.

Chronic viral hepatitis

Patients infected with hepatitis B or C viruses may become chronic carriers. These patients are at risk of continuing inflammation in the liver, leading to chronic hepatitis, cirrhosis, and ultimately, hepatocellular carcinoma.

Hepatitis B

All chronic carriers of hepatitis B virus have detectable surface antigen (HBsAg) in their peripheral blood. However, HBsAg-positive individuals can be subdivided further into those in whom HBeAg (a breakdown product of the viral core antigen) can be detected, and those with antibodies to this antigen, anti-HBe. HBeAg is a surrogate marker of active viral replication in hepatocytes. HBeAg-positive patients are considerably more infectious, and are at much greater risk of the long-term deleterious consequences of hepatitis B virus carriage, than are anti-HBe positive patients. For these reasons, therapy for chronic infection is targeted at those HBsAg carriers who are HBeAg positive.

Both standard interferon-α and pegylated formulations (p. 106–107) are beneficial in the treatment of chronic hepatitis B infection, but their action is immunomodulatory, rather than antiviral. Interferon enhances the expression of human leucocyte antigen (HLA) class I molecules on the surface of infected hepatocytes resulting in the efficient elimination of these cells by circulating cytotoxic T lymphocytes. This in turn reduces the amount of virus in the liver, and the production of infectious virions. HBeAg in the peripheral blood is replaced by anti-HBe.

A typical response of a hepatitis B virus carrier to interferon is shown in Fig. 27.1. At the onset of therapy, the patient is HBsAg and HBeAg positive, and has a raised alanine aminotransferase level, which indicates continuing liver cell damage. Some weeks after the initiation of interferon therapy, there is a marked rise in alanine aminotransferase. Paradoxically, this indicates a good therapeutic response, since it shows that hepatocytes now express sufficient HLA Class I molecules to allow recognition and destruction by cytotoxic lymphocytes. At the end of therapy, liver function returns to normal and the patient is now anti-HBe positive. Note that the patient remains HBsAg positive. Thus virus has not been completely eliminated, but the risk of ongoing liver damage is much reduced, and the patient is much less of an infection risk to sexual partners and family members. After a number of years, many patients do in fact eventually lose HBsAg.

Interferon is administered for up to 48 weeks. Even so, not all carriers respond to interferon. Those who have been carriers of the virus from birth (the vast majority world-wide) and patients who are immunocompromised (including those with HIV infection, in whom carriage of hepatitis B virus is common, as the routes of transmission of the two viruses are similar) respond poorly. In other patients, response rates are $>30\%$.

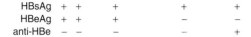

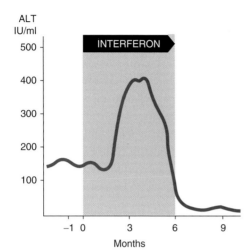

Fig. 27.1 Treatment of chronic hepatitis B infection with interferon showing the change in alanine aminotransferase (ALT) levels, loss of hepatitis B e antigen (HBeAg), and the appearance of antibody to HBe (anti-HBe). Hepatitis B surface antigen (HbsAg) is not eliminated.

New forms of therapy of chronic hepatitis B virus infection are becoming available. These include lamivudine, adefovir, tenofovir, and entecavir, which produce best results when combined with interferon. Lamivudine requires prolonged (>1 year) oral therapy to produce a 100-fold reduction in viral DNA titre, and histological improvement of liver biopsy appearance in more than 80% of patients. However, seroconversion rates to anti-HBe are much lower, at best 20%. Cessation of therapy leads to recurrence of viral replication. More prolonged therapy may improve the seroconversion rate, but this benefit must be weighed against the increased risk of the emergence of resistant virus. Adefovir and tenofovir are active against lamivudine-resistant mutants. Entecavir is the most potent agent to date.

Co-infection with HIV and hepatitis B virus is increasingly recognized and requires specialist management since agents such as lamivudine and tenofovir are active against both viruses and both infections require multidrug regimens for their management.

Another area in which these newer agents have shown promise is in the prophylaxis and treatment of hepatitis B positive patients undergoing liver and other forms of transplantation. There is a reduction in risk of severe disease in the case of a grafted liver and a reduced rate of virus reactivation associated with other procedures.

Hepatitis C

The relative success of interferon therapy in chronic hepatitis B infection led to trials of its use in chronic infection with hepatitis C virus. About 40–50% of such patients respond to a year's course of interferon, as judged by improvement in liver function and loss of viral RNA from serum. However, about half relapse when therapy is stopped, resulting in an overall cure rate of less than 20%. The mechanism of action of interferon in hepatitis C infection appears to be different from that in hepatitis B, as response is not accompanied by a rise in alanine aminotransferase levels.

Ribavirin therapy provides modest benefit in liver function in chronic hepatitis C disease. When combined with interferon, response rates are much better than with interferon alone, so that interferon monotherapy is no longer justifiable. The pegylated interferons are more potent and easier to administer and are now standard therapy.

Combination therapy with pegylated interferon and ribavirin is recommended for adults with moderate to severe chronic hepatitis C. Patients are assessed pretreatment for prognostic markers. A poor response is likely in: the presence of genotype 1 infection (hepatitis C virus exists in at least six distinct genotypes); high viral load; age > 40 years; pre-existing fibrosis on biopsy; and male sex. Such patients require prolonged treatment (48 weeks). Genotype 2 and 3 infections are more responsive to treatment; 24 weeks' therapy is generally sufficient.

The management of co-infection with HIV and hepatitis C virus is particularly challenging and requires specialist selection and supervision. The timing of treatment of hepatitis C in relation to the stage of HIV infection is crucial.

HIV infection

The management of HIV-infected patients has undergone enormous changes in the past few years. Advances in drug design and in understanding the replication cycle of HIV have led to the development of an increasing number of antiretroviral agents (see Table 7.1, p. 110). Moreover, application of molecular biological techniques allows accurate monitoring of the amount of HIV RNA in peripheral blood (viral load) in individual patients. Treatment regimens and management protocols are becoming ever more complex. In order to achieve some sort of standardization of clinical practice, bodies such as the British HIV Association publish consensus guidelines for antiretroviral treatment of HIV-seropositive individuals. Such is the pace of change that these guidelines need annual revision. It is nevertheless possible to discern some important underlying principles governing the appropriate use of antiretroviral therapy, although their detailed application may vary from place to place and over time.

Combination therapy

Initially zidovudine (AZT) was the only option available. However, resistance invariably develops through the selection of mutations in the error-prone reverse transcriptase gene, and AZT monotherapy loses its clinical benefit after about 6 months.

With the advent of more antiretroviral drugs, it became possible to model the treatment of HIV infection on that used for the treatment of tuberculosis: use of multiple agents to reduce the chances that the virus will become resistant to all of the drugs simultaneously. This principle has now been validated for a variety of combination therapies and has become the standard of care.

Triple drug combinations are highly effective in reducing viral load, both in degree and in duration of the effect. With the choice of agents including nucleoside analogues, non-nucleoside reverse transcriptase inhibitors, protease inhibitors, and a fusion inhibitor (Table 7.1, p. 110), there are numerous possible triple drug combinations. The continuing emergence of new agents will complicate this even further. It is clearly not possible to test each one of these combinations in full-scale clinical trials, but several regimens have proved to be highly effective. Such combination therapies are now collectively referred to as 'highly active antiretroviral therapy' (HAART).

Regimens recommended in the UK include two nucleoside reverse transcriptase inhibitors plus either a non-nucleoside reverse transcriptase inhibitor or a protease inhibitor. The reason for not selecting one drug of each category, which might appear intuitively to be the best idea, is to reserve one class of drugs for the time when initial therapy begins to fail, as it inevitably does. At this time, the virus present within the patient should at least be fully sensitive to all drugs of the unused class. In the absence of such 'class-sparing', the options for salvage therapy in the event of treatment failure are much reduced, as cross-resistance between drugs of the same class is common.

The exact choice of drugs for an individual patient depends on a number of variables. It cannot be assumed that virus in a patient who has received no previous antiretroviral therapy will be sensitive to all drugs, as the patient may have acquired a resistant strain. Such primary drug resistance now affects more than 10% of newly diagnosed patients in the UK. Moreover, adverse events are often unpredictable and regimens may need tailoring to individual patients. Clearly, the more drugs a patient takes, the greater the risk of adverse reactions. For example, there is particular concern about the long-term safety of protease inhibitors, owing to their effect on lipid metabolism.

Monitoring of therapy

For many years, the antiviral effect of drugs used in HIV-infected individuals could be determined only by measuring the level of circulating CD4-positive T cells as a surrogate marker of infection. The advent of viral load testing provides a much more direct measure of the efficacy of an antiviral drug. Viral load is of prognostic importance: the higher the load in an individual patient, the sooner that individual will develop AIDS and die. Thus the goal of antiretroviral therapy is to reduce viral load to undetectable levels. It is now possible routinely to detect as few as 50 copies of viral RNA per ml of plasma.

Failure of treatment for whatever reason can be detected by a rise in viral titres. Thus, long-term antiretroviral therapy is monitored by serial viral load measurements, and action taken if these levels rise. If failure is due to the emergence of resistance to one or more of the agents being taken, then appropriate changes in regimen should be instituted. It is possible to analyse the genome of the HIV present in a patient who is failing therapy, and identify which resistance mutations are present. Drug-resistance genotyping is expensive but has become integral to defining initial therapy and for identifying resistance arising during treatment. Comparative trials have shown that genotypic resistance testing confers a significant benefit on the virological response when choosing therapeutic alternatives.

In parallel with the reduction in viral load, CD4 counts rise, and there is at least a partial restoration of the previously damaged host immune system. As the immunodeficiency recedes, then the risk of those complications of HIV infection that define the acquired immune deficiency syndrome also recede. As a consequence, it may be possible to discontinue prophylaxis against infections such as pneumocystosis, toxoplasmosis, and cryptococcosis in patients responding successfully to HAART.

In addition to monitoring viral load and CD4, patients stabilized on HAART are reviewed every few months for clinical assessment, lipid analysis, and evidence of organ or bone marrow toxicity arising from treatment or complications of their HIV infection.

When to treat?

Given that there are now drugs available that can substantially decrease the viral load within an individual patient, and that this can be monitored, the question arises as to when antiretroviral therapy should be started. This decision is an important one. It requires commitment from the patient to take the medication for a prolonged period, usually for life. This may incur both physical and psychological morbidity, disadvantages that have to be weighed against the potential therapeutic benefits to be gained. At present, UK guidelines recommend starting therapy in any patient with symptomatic HIV infection or AIDS regardless of their viral load or CD4 count. In those who are asymptomatic the CD4 count is the major determinant for starting therapy. All those with counts < 200 cells/mm^3 are treated. Those with counts between 200 and 350 cells/mm^3 are evaluated further for viral load, rate of CD4 decline, evidence of coexisting conditions and patient preference. Currently, treatment is deferred for those with CD4 counts above 350 cells/mm^3. Evidence for long-term survival benefit of early treatment of primary HIV is lacking and this is no longer an indication for treatment.

Pregnancy

A special consideration is the use of antiretroviral drugs in pregnancy. There is compelling evidence that the risk of vertical transmission of HIV from mother to baby is proportional to the maternal viral load during pregnancy. Reduction of maternal viral load by use of antiretroviral agents significantly reduces the risk of transmission. Thus, all pregnant HIV carriers should be offered antiretroviral therapy regardless of whether or not they would otherwise qualify for such treatment. The choice of regimen will depend on the patient's past history of antiretroviral usage. Delivery should preferably be by caesarian section to further reduce the risk of virus transmission to the newborn. Breast feeding is not advised. In the UK, antiretroviral drugs are started between 28–32 weeks of pregnancy and during labour. The newborn is also treated for 6 weeks post-partum.

Importance of compliance

Drugs are only effective for as long as their concentration in the tissues is high enough. Failure to take the requisite regular doses of an antiviral drug leads to a fall in tissue levels, with a consequent risk of escape of the virus from inhibition of replication, and an increased likelihood of mutation to resistance. It is important, therefore, that patients adhere to the prescribed regimens. The more doses that are missed, the faster resistant virus will emerge.

Compliance is a significant problem, especially with multidrug regimens, in which some tablets should be taken with food and others on an empty stomach; some twice a day, others three or four times a day. By combining drugs in fixed dose formulations, compliance can be increased and is now the preferred treatment approach. Patients may also be on a variety of other agents; e.g. for prophylaxis against pneumocystis pneumonia or recurrent herpes simplex disease. Moreover, in any disease, and HIV infection is no exception, adherence to treatment is poorer in patients with symptom-free disease. Failure to take the tablets must always be considered as an explanation for a sudden rise in viral titre.

The complexity of HIV disease and its attendant complications, most notably of opportunistic infections (Chapter 28), require specialist manage-ment over many years. While HAART has substantially improved the survival and quality of life of those affected by HIV/AIDS, the disease remains incurable. New therapeutic approaches are needed, with novel modes of action and fewer side effects. This will remain the situation until an effective vaccine is developed, which despite an enormous research effort, remains an elusive goal.

HIV-positive patients are at risk of a wide range of serious infections. These are discussed in Chapter 28.

Other infections

Warts

Papillomavirus infections (warts) are amenable to physical (cryotherapy; surgery) and chemical (podophyllin and derivatives; salicylic acid) therapies. Interferons may have a place in the management of recalcitrant warts. About 50% of warts disappear following intralesional or intramuscular interferon, but they often recur. Topical application of imiquimod, a new imidazoquinoline that stimulates interferon and other cytokines, appears to be modestly effective.

Polyomavirus infections

Progressive multifocal leucoencephalopathy, a disease that occurs almost exclusively in HIV-positive and other immunosuppressed patients, is a manifestation of reactivation of a polyomavirus in the brain. Although it is of limited availability, the cytotoxic drug, cytosine arabinoside (Ara C) has been

normally sterile body site (bladder, vascular compartment) with the external environment.

The major features of immunosuppression associated with various malignant conditions are summarized in Table 28.2. Such patients are often cared for in high-dependency or intensive care facilities that provide opportunities for cross-infection and the acquisition of hospital-associated, and therefore more antibiotic-resistant, pathogens.

Microbial complications in the immunocompromised host

The variety of infections that may occur in the immunocompromised patient is extensive and arises from either exogenous (external source) or endogenous (host derived) micro-organisms. The distinction between exogenous and endogenous infections is not always clear-cut, since in hospital the bacterial flora of the skin and mucous membranes often alters.

In the case of virus infections, the herpes group predominates and may represent primary infection or reactivation of latent virus; these infections are often more severe than those in the immunocompetent host and carry the risk of dissemination. Adenovirus and para-influenza virus infections of the lung are also observed in profoundly neutropenic patients.

Fungal infections can be particularly severe. Candidosis of the mouth and upper gastrointestinal tract is particularly common and from time to time may be complicated by candidaemia, with spread to other organs. *Cryptococcus neoformans*, a yeast that was an uncommon cause of meningitis until the AIDS pandemic, occasionally complicates organ transplantation and malignant lymphoma.

Table 28.2 Examples of immunosuppressive states associated with an increased frequency or severity of infection according to altered host defences

Disease	Mucosal surfaces	Phagocytosis	Humoral immunity	CMI
Acute lymphoblastic leukaemia	+	++	−	+
Acute myeloblastic leukaemia	+	++	−	+
Chronic lymphocytic leukaemia	−	−	++	+
Hodgkin, non-Hodgkin lymphoma	−	−	−	+
Solid tumours	++	−	−	+
Multiple myeloma	−	−	++	−

CMI, cell-mediated immunity. −, association absent; +, definite association; ++, marked association.

Among the filamentous fungi, *Aspergillus* spp. are the most common pathogens. Their ubiquitous spores are normally harmless to the immuno-competent, but in the immunocompromised patient they can cause serious lung infection that may disseminate throughout the body. This risk is greatest in patients with profound neutropenia. Aspergillosis is not only difficult to treat but is also difficult to diagnose, especially in the early stages of infection.

Pneumocystis carinii (*jiroveci*) has emerged as the leading opportunistic infection complicating HIV infection. It primarily affects the lung where it produces a severe progressive pneumonia, which may be fatal unless treated early. Pneumocystosis may also occur in patients undergoing organ trans-plantation and in those with lymphoblastic leukaemia or malignant lym-phoma; profound impairment of cell-mediated immunity characterizes all these conditions. *P. carinii*, although a fungus, has a pattern of susceptibility to chemotherapeutic agents that is more in keeping with a protozoon. Other parasitic infections in the immunocompromised host include toxoplas-mosis and in endemic regions, leishmaniasis. There are also a variety of gut infections such as giardiasis, cryptosporidiosis, microsporidiosis, and strongyloidiasis. The latter can progress to a state of hyperinfection with extensive larval invasion of the body.

Principles of chemotherapeutic control

The vulnerability of the immunocompromised patient to infection has been emphasized. Not only is the range of possible infections broad, but, because of the state of immunosuppression, the presentation may be atypical and the course fulminant. A specific clinical and microbiological diagnosis can be difficult to establish; the therapeutic management of such patients is consequently based on a set of principles that has evolved to meet their particular needs.

It is essential that the patient is thoroughly examined at the earliest suspicion of infection. Particular attention should be paid to the skin, perineum, entry sites for catheters, the mouth, lungs, and abdomen. Appropriate microbiological samples should be collected and necessary radiographic investigations obtained. Timely biopsy of lymph nodes, bone marrow, cutaneous or intrapulmonary lesions is appropriate in selective cases. The approach to the chemotherapeutic management of the immuno-compromised patient is particularly well demonstrated in:

* patients with haematological malignancies undergoing cytotoxic chemo-therapy or bone marrow transplantation, especially during episodes of profound neutropenia;

* patients with AIDS;
* those with specific immunological defects such as hyposplenism.

Neutropenic patients

In the neutropenic patient infection can develop rapidly over a matter of hours, and if untreated can prove fatal. If fever above 38°C persists for 2 h or more, broad-spectrum antibiotic therapy should be administered promptly by the intravenous route. However, documentation of infection can be difficult: about 15% of infections will be documented by blood culture, a further 20% by other microbiological investigations, and a further 20% by clinical criteria. In the remainder, infection may only be strongly suspected without supporting clinical or laboratory evidence; non-microbial causes such as drug reactions, blood or platelet transfusions, or the underlying disease state may be responsible for the febrile episode.

Treatment regimens

The variety and relative frequency of bloodstream pathogens in the neutropenic patient are summarized in Table 28.3. There has been a striking increase in Gram-positive infections in recent years, which in part relates to the widespread use of vascular catheters for drug administration, as well as the selective pressure arising from the use of broad-spectrum antibiotics, notably β-lactam and quinolone agents.

In general the antibiotic regimens have been based on a combination of a β-lactam antibiotic and an aminoglycoside, which together are active against most of the likely pathogens. Among the β-lactam agents, a broad-spectrum cephalosporin such as ceftazidime has been most widely used, although the ureidopenicillin piperacillin, in combination with tazobactam, is also popular. An aminoglycoside such as gentamicin or amikacin is administered simultaneously since both are active against Gram-negative bacilli, including *Pseudomonas aeruginosa*. Some centres have adopted the use of a single agent such as ceftazidime or imipenem, but the combined regimen offers synergistic activity that may be useful, especially when dealing with serious *Ps. aeruginosa* bacteraemia. The increase in Gram-positive infections caused by staphylococci, enterococci, and viridans streptococci reflects a relative weakness in these regimens; as a result a glycopeptide, such as vancomycin or teicoplanin, may be needed, especially in patients who have recently undergone bone marrow transplantation in whom a neutropenic febrile episode can be particularly serious. However, increased use of glycopeptides is being accompanied by infections caused by glycopeptide-resistant enterococci.

Table 28.3 Distribution of bloodstream isolates complicating neutropenic states

Micro-organism	Approximate percentage
Gram-positive bacteria	
Staphylococcus epidermidis	28
Staph. aureus	10
Corynebacterium spp.	5
Streptococci	12
Gram-negative bacteria	
Gram-negative enteric bacilli	28
Pseudomonas aeruginosa	7
Others	7
Fungi	
Candida spp.	3

Candida infection is best treated with intravenous amphotericin B or caspofungin with the azole fluconazole as a reserve agent. Amphotericin B is a toxic drug and careful dosaging and monitoring of renal function is essential to avoid serious nephrotoxicity. Lipid formulations of amphotericin B are less nephrotoxic but much more expensive.

Cryptococcal yeast infections are managed with a combination of amphotericin with or without the addition of flucytosine (see Chapter 26, p. 372). Filamentous fungal infections, notably *Aspergillus* infection, are best treated with intravenous amphotericin B or voriconazole. An alternative agent for unresponsive disease is caspofungin.

Chemoprophylaxis

The seriousness of infections in the severely immunosuppressed neutropenic patient has led to the use of chemoprophylactic drug regimens, particularly in patients undergoing cytotoxic chemotherapy for haematological malignancies and in bone marrow transplant recipients. Regimens are directed at those micro-organisms likely to result in bacteraemic disease.

The varied choice of prophylactic regimen reflects different views on the pathogenesis of infection in these patients. One view is that oral, non-absorbable antibiotics are desirable in that their effect is confined to the gastrointestinal tract, which is the major source of invasive micro-organisms. These regimens are less widely used than in the past, but have included agents active against *Candida* spp., because of the frequency and severity of upper gastrointestinal candidosis, together with framycetin and colistin, which are non-absorbed agents. Other variations have included neomycin, colistin, and nystatin; or gentamicin, vancomycin, and nystatin. One important problem with these regimens is that their bitter taste leads to poor patient compliance. Moreover, evidence that they reduce the frequency and severity of bacteraemic infections has been difficult to obtain.

As an alternative to these regimens, other agents have been adopted which have systemic antibiotic effects. Co-trimoxazole has been widely used for its activity against many Gram-negative enteric bacilli and Gram-positive pathogens. It is also active against *P. carinii*. However, the emergence of drug-resistant strains, poor activity against *Ps. aeruginosa*, and the danger of bone marrow suppression in bone marrow recipients make this antifolate compound less than ideal.

Fluoroquinolones provide broad-spectrum activity, high potency, and a systemic antibiotic effect, with substantial drug concentrations within the gut. There is strong evidence to indicate that these drugs achieve a reduction in serious Gram-negative bacteraemia, although the relative weakness of the quinolones against Gram-positive pathogens has also been clearly demonstrated. Ciprofloxacin has been the most widely used agent. When given by mouth it provides a cost-effective approach in high-risk patients, especially those undergoing bone marrow transplantation.

Selective decontamination of the digestive tract

As well as patients rendered neutropenic by chemotherapy or disease, the ventilated patient on the intensive care unit is at considerable risk of infection, in particular from pneumonia from aspiration of oropharyngeal flora. One approach has been to use a topical antibiotic regimen, applied to the mouth in the form of paste and given in liquid form via a nasogastric tube into the stomach and hence the gastrointestinal tract. The aim is to suppress the flora of the gastrointestinal tract, which is largely made up of aerobic and anaerobic micro-organisms. One widely studied regimen is a combination of polymyxin, gentamicin, and amphotericin B, often supplemented for the first few days with intravenous cefotaxime. The pathogens targeted by this regimen include *Staphylococcus aureus*, *Escherichia coli*, *Proteus* spp., *Klebsiella* spp., and *Candida* spp., which are among the more common causes of infection in such patients. Studies have shown a reduction in bacterial counts in the mouth, stomach, and colon. There is also evidence that nosocomial pneumonia can be reduced. This is more readily achievable, in young, relatively fit patients who have sustained major trauma than in the elderly or those with chronic lung disease. Among other populations of ventilated patients the cost–benefit of this procedure in terms of reduced mortality and length of stay in hospital has proved difficult to establish.

AIDS

The clinical impact of HIV infection lies in its persistent nature and the accompanying progressive immunodeficiency which gives rise to a range of complicating infections and malignancies. These target many organs as well as producing systemic illness. Table 28.4 summarizes the more important complicating infections.

In contrast to their effects in the immunocompetent host, these infections often present atypically and with heightened severity. Furthermore, many of the infections recur after treatment in those with advanced HIV disease. Thus, in the HIV-infected patient the initial course of treatment must be more intensive than in the immunocompetent host, and for many conditions long-term suppressive therapy is needed to prevent relapse. In addition, by controlling the underlying HIV infection, the frequency and severity of opportunistic infections can be reduced, as well as the risk of recurrent opportunistic infection.

The introduction of 'highly active antiretroviral therapy' (HAART), in which three-drug regimens of two nucleoside analogues with a protease inhibitor or a non-nucleoside reverse transcriptase inhibitor are used, has permitted cessation of primary prophylaxis against *P. carinii* in selected patients. These regimens are discussed in Chapter 27. They are generally well tolerated and, provided the patient is compliant with the medication, have a major impact on the quality of life. Although they all act in a suppressive manner to delay disease progression, none is curative.

The chemotherapeutic approach to selected opportunistic infections is discussed in order to emphasize the principles and associated problems that arise.

Pneumocystis carinii (P. jiroveci)

Among the many opportunistic infections that complicate HIV infection, *P. carinii* predominates. The primary site of infection is the lung. Clinical disease represents reactivation of endogenous infection usually acquired in childhood. Typical symptoms include progressive shortness of breath with or without a relatively unproductive cough, progressive hypoxaemia, and diffuse

Table 28.4 Common opportunist pathogens complicating HIV disease

Site	Micro-organism
Gastrointestinal tract	*Cryptosporidium parvum*
	Salmonella enterica serotypes
	Mycobacterium avium complex
	Cytomegalovirus
	Herpes simplex
	Candida spp.
Respiratory tract	*Pneumocystis carinii (jiroveci)*
	Streptococcus pneumoniae
	Mycobacterium tuberculosis
	Cytomegalovirus
Central nervous system	*Toxoplasma gondii*
	Cryptococcus neoformans
	Cytomegalovirus
	Herpes simplex
	Varicella zoster
	JC polyoma virus

bilateral chest radiograph infiltrates. The diagnosis has been greatly facilitated by the availability of a fluorescent antibody to *P. carinii*, which can be applied to expectorated sputum or to a saline lavage obtained by bronchoscopy.

The treatment of choice is high-dose co-trimoxazole, by mouth or intravenously, for 3 weeks. The risk of hypersensitivity to the sulphonamide component is greatly increased in HIV disease and alternative regimens, such as intravenous pentamidine or oral atovaquone, or a combination of clindamycin and primaquine may be necessary. Intravenous trimetrexate has also been used in patients intolerant of or unresponsive to other drugs.

Once the patient has recovered it is necessary to continue with life-long prophylaxis with low-dose co-trimoxazole. Alternative agents that can be used in those intolerant of the standard regimens include dapsone, clindamycin, and primaquine. Nebulized pentamidine given once monthly as an aerosol inhalation provides another choice. In view of the seriousness of *P. carinii* pneumonia, patients with HIV infection are now offered primary prophylaxis when their CD4 lymphocyte counts fall below 200/µl in order to prevent infection. The choice of agent and frequency of administration is the same as for secondary prophylaxis.

Toxoplasmosis

The protozoon *Toxoplasma gondii* can cause serious disease in people with HIV infection. This may occur as a primary infection, although it more usually represents reactivation of dormant parasites. The disease presents most frequently as a space-occupying lesion of the brain with focal neurological features. The diagnosis is based on clinical suspicion and computed tomography scan. Serodiagnosis is difficult. The presence of tachyzoites in brain biopsy is confirmatory. However, it is more usual to carry out a trial of chemotherapy in the first instance since this can avoid potentially dangerous neurosurgery.

Toxoplasmosis is treated with pyrimethamine and sulfadiazine in high dosage for 6 weeks before reducing to a maintenance dose. This regimen often results in bone marrow suppression or is complicated by an allergic skin eruption. Alternative drugs include high-dose clindamycin or the azalide azithromycin, which also exhibits useful activity. The principles of treatment are similar to those for controlling *P. carinii* pneumonia in that initial control is followed by lifelong maintenance therapy. There is evidence that co-trimoxazole given as prophylaxis for *P. carinii* may also be suppressive for toxoplasmosis.

Cytomegalovirus infection

Cytomegalovirus infection is extremely common. In those with HIV infection, reactivation is associated with a range of manifestations, which may involve the gastrointestinal tract, lung, liver, and in particular the eye, where a progressive retinopathy may lead to loss of vision or total blindness. Treatment with ganciclovir, foscarnet, or cidofovir is suppressive but not curative (see Chapter 27).

Mycobacteriosis

Patients with HIV infection are at increased risk of mycobacterial infection. This may be newly acquired but is more usually the result of endogenous reactivation as cell-mediated immunity steadily declines. *Mycobacterium tuberculosis* is the infecting organism, but disease may present atypically owing to altered host immunity. In many parts of the world drug-resistant tuberculosis has emerged as an important problem, and there have been instances of spread within prisons and hospitals (see p. 353). Where there is good evidence for previous tuberculosis, chemoprophylaxis with isoniazid is recommended for 1–2 years.

Infection with organisms of the *Mycobacterium avium* complex is a common problem in patients with AIDS. Disease presents with fever, sweats, weight loss, and diarrhoea. Patients are frequently bacillaemic and have high bacterial loads within the gut and bone marrow. The organisms are extremely resistant to conventional antituberculosis regimens and a combination of clarithromycin with rifabutin and ethambutol is recommended. Response to treatment may, unfortunately, be short-lived. Attempts have therefore been directed at preventing disease with rifabutin, alone or in combination with azithromycin.

Hyposplenism

The spleen is an important site of host defences, rich in lymphoid follicles and phagocytic cells. In its absence the patient is at increased risk of infection, including fulminating bacteraemia. Apart from splenectomy, a variety of medical conditions can cause hyposplenism. These include hereditary conditions such as sickle cell anaemia and hereditary spherocytosis. The risk of serious infections is greatest in early childhood but declines with age, although the risk remains throughout life. Among the fulminant infections are those caused by *Streptococcus pneumoniae, Haemophilus influenzae, Esch. coli, Neisseria meningitidis,* and a rare pathogen of man, *Capnocytophaga canimorsus.* Hyposplenic or asplenic patients should be alerted to their increased risk and recommended to seek early medical attention in the presence of symptoms suggestive of severe infection. Immunization against pneumococcal infections is possible in those over 2 years of age and is the best form of prevention. Likewise, children should be immunized against *H. influenzae and* group C meningococcal infection. Long-term chemoprophylaxis with phenoxymethylpenicillin (penicillin V) is of proven benefit in children with sickle cell disease. However, the additional benefit of life-long prophylaxis in those who have been actively immunized is marginal. Compliance with lifelong penicillin V prophylaxis is a further problem, as is the steady increase in resistance to penicillin among pneumococci, especially in parts of Europe and North America.

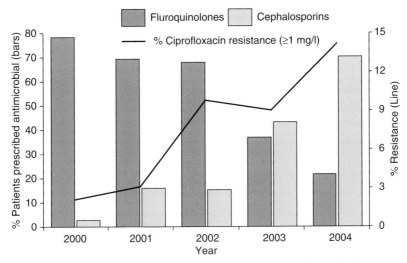

Fig. 29.2 Relative prescribing of cephalosporins and fluoroquinolones for the treatment of gonorrhoea in genito-urinary medicine clinics in England and Wales, and prevalence of resistance to ciprofloxacin, 2000–2004.

Table 29.2 Prevalence of resistance in *N. gonorrhoeae* isolates from laboratories in England and Wales, 2003 and 2004

Antimicrobial agent (breakpoint concentration)	Prevalence of resistance (%)		P value for change 2003 versus 2004
	2003	2004	
Penicillin (≥1 mg/l or β-lactamase positive)	9.7	11.2	P = 0.5
Tetracycline (≥2 mg/l)	38.2	44.5	P < 0.005
Ciprofloxacin (≥ 1 mg/l)	9.0	14.1	P = 0.01
Azithromycin (≥ mg/l)	0.9	1.8	P < 0.05
Spectinomycin (≥ 128 mg/l)	0	0.2	N/A
Ceftriaxone (≥0.125 mg/l)	0	0	N/A
Cefixime (≥ 0.25 mg/l)	0	0	N/A

Data from gonococcal antimicrobial resistance surveillance programme (GRASP). Available at: http://www.hpa.org.uk/infections/topics_az/hiv_and_sti/sti-gonorrhoea/publications/ GRASP_2004_Annual_Report.pdf

prolonged antibiotics. Non-genital gonococcal infection also requires more than a single dose of penicillin to achieve cure (see below).

Non-gonococcal (non-specific) urethritis or cervicitis

After penicillin became available for the treatment of gonorrhoea it was evident that some treated individuals still had symptoms of urethritis or cervicitis or both. The terms non-specific or non-gonococcal urethritis were used to refer to such cases or when gonococci could not be demonstrated despite symptoms. It is now clear that most of these infections are caused by *C. trachomatis*, an obligate intracellular pathogen that is difficult to diagnose, requiring culture in cell lines. Indeed, numbers of *C. trachomatis* sexually transmitted infections now far exceed cases of gonorrhoea in most developed countries. Of great concern, *C. trachomatis* is a major cause of pelvic inflammatory disease in women (see below), which can lead to infertility. Some cases of non-gonococcal urethritis are probably due to ureaplasmas or mycoplasmas, but as these cell wall deficient bacteria may be found in some healthy individuals diagnosis of infection is difficult and not routinely practised. *Trichomonas vaginalis*, herpesvirus, urinary tract infection, and local causes such as trauma also account for some cases of urethritis/cervicitis.

C. trachomatis infection can now be detected by nucleic acid amplification tests on cervical or urethral swabs and, because of the greatly improved sensitivity of this approach compared with culture or enzyme immunoassays, on urine. The availability of urine testing means that cumbersome invasive sampling, and internal examination in females, is no longer required for the detection of chlamydia infection. Furthermore, screening of urine samples from young sexually active people, particularly those frequently changing sexual partners, is increasingly used to detect subclinical chlamydia infection.

Tetracyclines, especially doxycycline, given for at least 7 days are effective. Failure of therapy occurs and may reflect poor compliance or re-infection. A single dose of azithromycin is as effective as 1–2 weeks of tetracycline therapy and clearly overcomes compliance problems. It is considerably more expensive than tetracyclines, but improved overall compliance and efficacy may mean that it is cost-effective. Erythromycin can also be used for 1–2 weeks, but the relatively poor gastrointestinal side effect profile does not encourage compliance. Genuine relapses of infection are possibly due to latent phase chlamydial infection. Antimicrobial resistance is thought to be rare, but as routine culture and susceptibility testing of *C. trachomatis* is not practised limited data are available. Chlamydiae are eukaryotic cells, and although these bacteria lack a peptidoglycan cell wall, ampicillin and

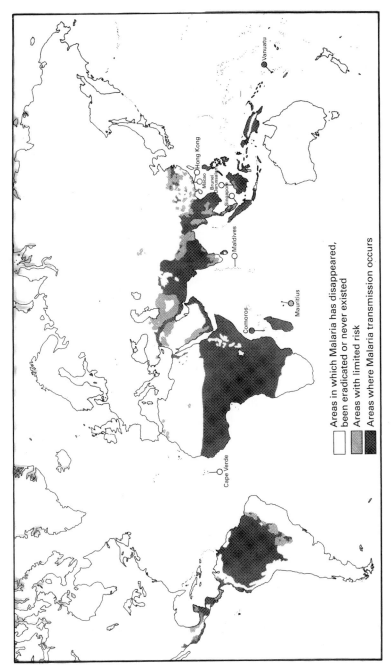

Fig. 30.1 Distribution of malaria 2004. Reproduced from http://www.who.int/malaria with permission from The World Health Organisation.

of the tropical world, particularly in parts of Africa where many children die of falciparum malaria before they reach the age of 5.

Acute malaria

After the Second World War chloroquine replaced the traditional remedy quinine as the drug of choice for the treatment of acute malaria. These agents are active against the blood forms of the parasite, which is important in the symptomatic stage of the disease when rapidly dividing schizonts cause red cell lysis; it is particularly important in falciparum malaria when infected erythrocytes block small cerebral blood vessels to give rise to the rapidly fatal form of cerebral malaria. In such cases urgent parenteral therapy is necessary in spite of the hazards of infusion.

In its time, chloroquine revolutionized the treatment and prophylaxis of malaria, but extensive use led to the appearance of resistant strains of *Plasmodium falciparum* in most areas in which the parasite occurs. Many chloroquine-resistant strains are also resistant to alternative drugs such as the combinations of pyrimethamine with sulphonamides or dapsone. Surprisingly for such an ancient remedy, resistance to quinine remains quite rare and the drug has returned to favour for severe falciparum malaria. Because of the possibility of reduced susceptibility to quinine, treatment with doxycycline or clindamycin, antibacterial antibiotics that also exhibit antimalarial activity, is also usually included. Species of *Plasmodium* other than *P. falciparum* generally retain susceptibility to chloroquine and it still remains the drug of choice in benign tertian and quartan malarias.

Derivatives of a Chinese herbal remedy, qinghaosu (artemisinin) are increasingly being used for the treatment of malaria in the tropics. Although animal experiments revealed a potential for neurotoxicity, extensive trials and increasing clinical experience have shown these compounds to be relatively safe and their future as antimalarial agents appears progressively more secure. Various formulations, including artesunic acid (artesunate), artemotil (β-arteether) and artemether are used for intravenous or intramuscular administration. Artesunate can also be given by mouth. Suppository formulations are also available and are particularly useful in children. Artemisinin derivatives are now being recommended as the drugs of choice in uncomplicated falciparum malaria; since they are more rapidly effective than any other drug, they are also now being used as an alternative to quinine in severe forms of the disease. Because of the risk of encouraging the development of resistance, it is strongly recommended that artemisinin derivatives should be used together with other antimalarial drugs: artemether with lumefantrine can be given orally if the patient is able to

Babesiosis

Infections in splenectomized patients, usually caused by *Babesia divergens*, is life-threatening and requires urgent treatment, but experience is limited. There is evidence that the combination of clindamycin and quinine is useful, but exchange transfusion may also be needed. Infection with *B. microti* in previously healthy persons is usually self-limiting, but clindamycin and quinine can be used if therapy is warranted. The combination of azithromycin and atovaquone has also been used with success.

Other protozoan infections

Treatment of infection with intestinal protozoa such as *Isospora belli*, *Cyclospora cayetanensis*, and various microsporidia is poorly defined, although co-trimoxazole (isosporiasis and cyclosporiasis) and albendazole (microsporidiosis) have been successfully used. In patients with AIDS these opportunist infections usually remit when the CD4 lymphocyte count improves on antiretroviral therapy.

Treatment of infection with the flagellate protozoon *Trichomonas vaginalis* is considered in Chapter 29 (p. 418).

Nematode infections

Filariasis

Well over 200 million people harbour filarial worms and in some areas of the tropics nearly the whole population is infected. Diagnosis is made by microscopical demonstration of the larval forms (microfilariae) in blood or, in the special case of *Onchocerca volvulus*, in superficial shavings of skin. Some of the blood microfilariae exhibit a curious periodicity in that they are found in peripheral blood during only the day (*Loa loa*) or the night (*Wuchereria bancrofti*). *Brugia malayi* (which is restricted to South-east Asia) usually exhibits a less complete nocturnal periodicity. *W. bancrofti* and *B. malayi* cause a clinically identical condition (lymphatic filariasis) sometimes resulting in elephantiasis owing to blockage of the lymphatics of the lower trunk. The clinical syndrome is due to a variety of factors depending on degree of exposure and host reaction to the worms, and in any area a small proportion will have gross elephantiasis. Often by this stage the disease may be 'burnt out' and an anthelminthic may do little to improve the patient's condition, for which surgical and supportive measures are all that is left. *O. volvulus*, the causative parasite of river blindness, affects large numbers of people in west Africa and central America. As with the other filariases, many infected persons exhibit only minor symptoms such as skin swelling and itching.

The introduction of ivermectin and albendazole has revolutionized the therapy of filarial infections. These relatively non-toxic drugs are now preferred for the treatment of onchocerciasis and lymphatic filariasis respectively. One of the benefits of their use is that reactions to treatment are a good deal milder than with the traditional drug, diethylcarbamazine, although ivermectin sometimes gives rise to an encephalopathy in individuals co-infected with *Loa loa*. Ivermectin is administered as a single oral dose, which is repeated annually in endemic areas. Mass treatment with ivermectin, together with vector control, has virtually eradicated onchocerciasis in some districts, and there are hopes that lymphatic filariasis will be similarly controlled with a combination of ivermectin and albendazole. The manufacturers of these drugs are providing them free for control programmes in countries where the diseases are endemic.

Toxocariasis

Infection with the dog roundworm *Toxocara canis* may cause a condition known as visceral larva migrans, which may result in serious eye infection usually presenting as a visual loss in childhood. Although not a common disease it is found worldwide and is probably under-recognized. The larvae of the worm migrate to the retina, setting up an inflammatory response. Treatment with diethylcarbamazine has been recommended but hypersensitivity reactions may require steroids to be given as well. Albendazole (or mebendazole) appears to offer an effective and less toxic alternative.

Intestinal nematode infections

Single doses of the common agents such as piperazine, levamisole, and pyrantel pamoate give acceptable cure rates. Table 30.1 shows the differential activity of these and the oral benzimidazole derivatives, which have a broader spectrum and have largely superseded them, but are more expensive. Among benzimidazoles, albendazole exhibits the best broad-spectrum anthelminthic activity. Tiabendazole (thiabendazole) is often poorly tolerated and is best avoided if possible.

In warm countries with poor water supplies and inadequate methods of sewage disposal re-infection with intestinal worms is almost inevitable, though simple health education advice on preventive measures may be valuable.

and axillae, or the genitalia after sexual contact. The mite burrows into the skin to form tunnels, which are diagnostic of the condition. There is often a more generalized hypersensitivity rash away from the area of penetration. All areas are itchy and scratching can lead to secondary bacterial infections, including impetigo.

Benzyl benzoate is effective, but is unpleasant to use, frequently causes irritation, and is not recommended for children. This has led to the use of the pyrethroid, permethrin, and the organophosphorus compound, malathion. Malathion should not be used repeatedly over a short period. Lindane (hexachlorocyclohexane; now discontinued in the UK) is strongly suspected to be carcinogenic and should not be used.

The key to treatment of scabies is careful, complete application of the lotion and reapplication if hands have been washed during the period the insecticide is in contact with the skin. The whole body should be covered, with particular attention to hands, fingers, and nails, and left to act overnight, or preferably 24 h.

Immunocompromised patients, such as those with HIV and old people, may develop a very heavy infestation that may crust over—so-called Norwegian scabies. Oral treatment with ivermectin has been tried with some success.

Lice

The most common infestation in the developed world is due to head lice (*Pediculus capitis*). The adult lice pass from person to person during close contact and attach their eggs (nits) to hair. The infestation may spread in schools and the community and total eradication is probably impossible, though most people develop resistance to re-infection.

There is no ideal insecticide for treatment of head lice. Among agents that are used, resistance to permethrin, phenothrin, and malathion occurs; carbaryl is usually effective, but there are fears about possible toxicity. 'Wet combing', by passing a fine-tooth comb through hair that has just been washed with conditioner, is useful, but should be repeated two to three times a week for several weeks to remove all the lice. Various herbal shampoos, such as tea tree oil, have advocates, but there is little evidence that they are effective. Shaving the head is a drastic measure, which is not recommended.

Pubic lice (*Phthirus pubis*; 'crab' lice) hold tenaciously to pubic hair, but can also be found on the head and eyelashes. Aqueous preparations of insecticides, such as malathion, should be applied overnight to all parts of the body. They are generally easier to treat than head lice, but it is important to find and treat sexual contacts and to remember that other sexually transmitted infections may be present.

Further reading

World Health Organization. *WHO Model Prescribing Information: drugs used in parasitic disease.* 2nd edition. WHO, Geneva, 1995.

World Health Organization. *Guidelines for the Treatment of Malaria.* WHO, Geneva, 2006. Available at: http://www.who.int/malaria/docs/TreatmentGuidelines2006.pdf

Chapter 31

Topical use of antimicrobial agents

The concept of applying drugs directly to clinical lesions is appealing: problems of absorption and pharmacokinetics do not apply and agents too toxic for systemic use may be safely applied to skin or mucous membranes. The major drawback is that, even in the most superficial skin lesion, there may be areas inaccessible to a topical approach. Furthermore, collections of pus may prevent the agent reaching the infecting organisms and for this reason the management of any abscess includes drainage of pus.

Although skin, the largest and most accessible organ of the body, is the most obvious target for topical antimicrobial agents, other sites are available for this approach to therapy: the mucous membranes of the mouth and vagina, and the external surfaces of eyes and ears. Direct application of antibiotics into normally sterile sites, such as joints, spinal fluid, or the urinary bladder, or instillation into surgical wounds prior to suture, may also be considered as a form of topical therapy, but will not be specifically dealt with in this chapter. Application of topical agents to mucous membranes or damaged skin may lead to considerable systemic absorption and the possibility of systemic toxicity should be borne in mind.

The chief reasons for using topical antimicrobial agents are:

* to achieve high drug concentrations at the site of infection;
* to treat trivial infections where use of a systemic drug is unjustified;
* to prevent infection in a susceptible site (e.g. burns);
* to enable the use of agents that are too toxic for systemic use;
* cost: topical agents are generally cheaper than systemic drugs.

Antiseptics

Disinfectant is a general term for chemicals that can destroy vegetative micro-organisms; those disinfectants that are sufficiently non-injurious to skin and exposed tissues to be used topically are called antiseptics. In order to achieve adequate antimicrobial activity, high concentrations of antiseptics are required and this serves to distinguish them from antibiotics in Waksman's original sense of 'substances produced by micro-organisms antagonistic to the growth or life of others in high dilution'. In many cases, true antibiotics are used topically in high concentration and might thus be classed as antiseptics. In fact, antiseptics and antibiotics are often used in exactly the same situations in dermatological practice and there has been some difference of opinion as to which class of agent to use in, for example, the treatment of infected ulcers or wounds. Antiseptics are usually cheaper and have the advantage that bacterial resistance rarely, if ever, develops. Preparations commonly employed include chlorhexidine, cetrimide, iodo-phors (non-irritant iodine complexes), triclosan, and solutions liberating hypochlorite, such as Eusol or Dakin's solution.

Some concern has been expressed about the effect on tissue viability of many chemicals applied directly. There is some evidence in vitro of a direct toxic effect on epidermal cells and white blood cells of many antiseptics at concentrations well below those used topically.

Methods of application

Drugs that are dissolved in aqueous solutions (lotions) have the disadvantage of running off the skin and cooling it by evaporation. This method of delivering antimicrobial agents to the site of infection is inefficient and not often used, except as ear or eye drops. For use in eye infections, frequent application on to the cornea and conjunctiva is necessary, because the drug is only in contact for a short time and much of the active component runs down the cheek as an expensive tear! The value of aqueous preparations resides mainly in their irrigant and cleansing action and much of the therapeutic success may be due to these properties.

It is usual to apply drugs to the skin in a fat base, as either an oil and water cream, or a largely lipid ointment. Drug solubility affects the achievable concentration in each component, and availability at the lesion depends on diffusion from the applicant and absorption from the skin. Antibiotics that are lipid soluble and freely diffusible, for example fusidic acid, are at an advantage in this respect.

Sticky ointments may remain in contact with the infected site for a considerable time and application may be needed only once daily, but this obviously depends on the frequency of washing or removal of dressings.

Some of the commonly used topical preparations are listed in Table 31.1. Many of the formulations designed for topical use contain

Table 31.1 Commonly used topical antimicrobial agents for skin infections. The numerous topical antiseptics available are omitted

Infection	Agent	Application	Comments
Bacterial	Chloramphenicol[a]	Ointment	Very broad spectrum
	Clindamycin[a]	Ointment	Used for acne
	Erythromycin[a]	Ointment	Used for acne
	Fusidic acid[a]	Ointment	Only active against *Staph. aureus* and *Str. pyogenes*
	Gentamicin[a]	Cream/ointment	Ototoxic and nephrotoxic if used over large areas of broken skin
	Metronidazole[a]	Gel	Used in rosacea and acne
	Mupirocin	Ointment	Macrogol-based ointment unsuitable for nasal application
	Neomycin	Cream/ointment/powder	Often combined with gramicidin or bacitracin and/or polymyxin B. Ototoxic and nephrotoxic if used over large areas of broken skin
	Polymyxins[a]	Ointment/ powder	Nephrotoxic and neurotoxic if used over large areas of broken skin
	Silver sulfadiazine (sulphonamide)	Cream	May cause sensitization
	Tetracycline[a]	Ointment/cream/drops	Broad-spectrum; resistance common
Fungal	Imidazoles (clotrimazole, etc.)	Cream/powder	For dermatophyte or yeast skin infections but ineffective against nail infections
	Nystatin (and other polyenes)	Cream	For dermatophyte or yeast skin infections but ineffective against nail infections
	Tioconazole and amorolfine	Nail lacquer/cream	For limited dermatophyte nail infections
Viral	Aciclovir[a] and penciclovir[a]	Ointment/cream	Antiviral agents; for use on herpes lesions
	Idoxuridine	Ointment/drops	

[a]Compounds that are also used systemically.

combinations of antimicrobial agents. Mixtures are intended to cover a wide antibacterial spectrum and to be compatible.

Choice

The results of laboratory tests may be helpful if adequate specimens are sent to the laboratory, but swabbing chronic ulcers or other skin wounds is not helpful (Chapter 23). Frequently, colonizing microbes are isolated from the surface of deep lesions leaving the true underlying pathogen undetected. The clinician must be careful not to use a battery of anti-microbials to treat harmless commensals colonizing an unoccupied niche. The golden rule is 'treat the patient, not the wound'.

Conventional antimicrobial sensitivity testing is often irrelevant because susceptibility of organisms to antiseptics can usually be assumed. Moreover, laboratory criteria of susceptibility to antibiotics usually apply to systemic use, not the high concentrations achievable by topical application. Never-theless, complete resistance in laboratory tests is a contra-indication to use of a particular agent. Regular monitoring of hospital patients with large skin lesions, such as ulcers and burns, is useful to determine the nature and prevalence of resistant organisms, as well as the extent of cross-infection.

Choice, if not based on microbiological evidence, must include agents active against all likely pathogens. Topical antiseptics and hydroxyquinolines are to be preferred to antibiotics on microbiological grounds of avoidance of resistance, but many users prefer antibiotics because it is claimed that a quicker response is generally obtained. Tetracyclines are often recommended by clinicians, but not by microbiologists, who point to the prevalence of tetracycline resistance and the readiness with which such prevalence increases under selective pressure. Combinations of antibiotics, such as bacitracin and neomycin, or bacitracin, neomycin, and polymyxin are often used, and a corticosteroid is sometimes added for good measure. These antibiotics are not usually used for systemic therapy, so possible problems of com-promising the activity of systemically useful agents by encouraging the emergence of resistance are minimized (see below). Nevertheless, it should be remembered that the topical use of neomycin might generate strains of bacteria cross-resistant to other aminoglycosides such as gentamicin.

One antibiotic, mupirocin (pseudomonic acid), has been marketed solely for topical use. The spectrum of activity of this agent is virtually restricted to Gram-positive cocci. Mupirocin is unsuitable for systemic use since it is quickly metabolized in the body (see p. 51). It has a unique mode of action (on protein synthesis) and cross-resistance is not a problem.

fungal infections of toenails may not completely clear even after a year's treatment with griseofulvin, despite susceptibility of the infecting fungus. In such cases terbinafine (p. 72) may be successful. Topical treatment with amorolfine or tioconazole, which are formulated to penetrate nails, are less effective than terbinafine.

Thrush responds in most cases to an appropriate antifungal agent, applied topically (e.g. nystatin or an imidazole), but precipitating factors, such as diabetes or antibiotic therapy, must also be corrected if they are present. If there is clinical evidence for invasive infection, as, for example, *Candida* oesophagitis, appropriate systemic drugs, such as amphotericin B, 5-fluorocytosine, fluconazole, ketoconazole, or itraconazole must be added.

Disadvantages of topical therapy

Topical therapy is not without its hazards. Although the direct toxic effects of drugs given systemically are reduced, exposed tissues and mucous membranes offer a fairly efficient site for drug absorption. For example, aminoglycoside ototoxicity has been reported following local application of neomycin, especially in the newborn. A more frequently observed effect is sensitization to the agent so that subsequent use of the drug, either topically or parenterally, produces a hypersensitivity reaction. Penicillin, in particular, is prone to sensitize the host and because of possible anaphylactic reactions it is not advisable to use any β-lactam antibiotic on the skin. A further hazard of topical therapy is that local irritation may lead to a delay in wound healing, even though the actual infection is controlled.

Superinfection with resistant bacteria or with fungi is a common consequence of using any topical antibiotic for a prolonged period. Widespread use of one particular agent will lead to a larger reservoir of resistant organisms and the possibility of cross-infection. This is particularly likely to occur in burns units and dermatology wards, where there are many patients with large open skin lesions. Prevention of infection and cross-infection by aseptic methods is desirable, but often difficult in practice.

Of equal concern is the development of bacterial resistance during therapy. It has been shown that topical neomycin can select resistant *Staphylococcus epidermidis* strains, which can transfer resistance to *Staph. aureus* on the skin. The emergence of gentamicin-resistant *Ps. aeruginosa* and coliforms has been associated with topical use of that aminoglycoside, particularly on leg ulcers. In some instances the resistance is plasmid mediated. In this manner, topical agents select multiresistant organisms, which may subsequently cause systemic infection in the patient or, by cross-infection, others.

Tetracycline eye drops select for tetracycline resistant bacteria in the mouth flora when used for mass population treatment of trachoma. The explanation is likely to be that medications administered to the eye can readily reach the nasopharynx via the naso-lachrymal duct. Selection of resistant bacteria is the most powerful argument against the indiscriminate use of topical antibiotics, and since antiseptics lack this disadvantage they are to be preferred wherever possible.

Chapter 32

Postscript: The development and marketing of antimicrobial drugs

Until the 1990s, most effort towards the discovery and development of new antimicrobial agents was expended on compounds active against bacteria, but the demands of the market place have caused the emphasis to shift. Of 67 new antimicrobial agents released on to the UK market between 1990 and 2004 (Table 32.1), only 26 were antibacterial agents, and antiviral agents now represent the largest single group of newly marketed compounds. Moreover, nearly all new antibacterial agents are chemically modified variants of existing compounds, whereas entirely new classes of antiviral agent are starting to emerge.

The progress of a new antibiotic from discovery to marketing is outlined in Fig 32.1. When a new antimicrobial drug is discovered or invented, the first indications of its activity and spectrum are usually gleaned from fairly simple in-vitro inhibition tests against a few common representative organisms. Organisms with special growth requirements, such as chlamydiae, mycobacteria, and mycoplasmas are usually excluded from such primary screening.

In-vitro screening tests will not detect potentially useful activity if in-vivo metabolism of the compound is a prerequisite for the antimicrobial effect (e.g. Prontosil; see Historical introduction); nor will such tests reveal agents that might modify microbial cells sufficiently to render them non-virulent or susceptible to host defences, without actually preventing

Table 32.1 Newly marketed antimicrobial agents in 3-year periods 1990–2004 (UK)

Period	Antibacterial agents	Antiviral agents	Antifungal agents	Antiparasitic agents
1990–1992	10	1	2	2
1993–1995	7	4	1	1
1996–1998	3	9	1	1
1999–2001	3	8	0	1
2002–2004	3	8	2	0

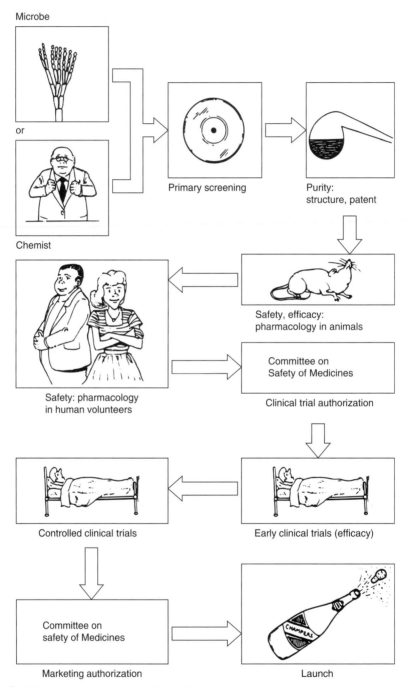

Microbe

or

Chemist

Primary screening

Purity: structure, patent

Safety, efficacy: pharmacology in animals

Safety: pharmacology in human volunteers

Committee on Safety of Medicines

Clinical trial authorization

Controlled clinical trials

Early clinical trials (efficacy)

Committee on safety of Medicines

Marketing authorization

Launch

Fig. 32.1 Progress of a new antibiotic from discovery to marketing

their growth. Furthermore, conventional laboratory culture media occasionally contain substances that interfere with the activity of certain antimicrobial compounds, which may consequently go undetected.

Despite these difficulties, in-vitro screening offers an extremely simple and generally effective way of detecting antimicrobial activity, which has yielded a rich harvest of therapeutically useful compounds over the years. In contrast, the rational design of antimicrobial agents that can disable vulnerable stages of microbial development has not been very fruitful so far, although new techniques of genomics, molecular modelling, and combinatorial chemistry offer the prospect that this might change in the future. Indeed, some of the new antiviral agents have been developed by targeting specific viral processes.

Development of new compounds

Compounds that pass the initial screening tests must be made available in sufficient quantities and in sufficiently pure form to enable preliminary tests of toxicity and efficacy to be carried out in laboratory animals, and more extensive and precise in-vitro tests to be performed. Pilot-stage production usually presents little problem, although considerable difficulties may be experienced in scaling up production at a later date, when relatively large quantities of highly purified drug are needed for clinical trials and subsequent marketing.

Animal tests of toxicity, pharmacology, and efficacy are an indispensable part of the development of any new drug, but they also have certain limitations. Idiosyncratic reactions may suggest toxicity in a compound that would be safe for human use or, more importantly, adverse reactions peculiar to the human subject may go undetected. The pharmacological handling of the drug may be vastly different from that encountered in the human subject. As regards efficacy testing, animals have important limitations in that experimental infections seldom correspond to the supposedly analogous human condition, either anatomically or in the relationship of treatment to the natural history of the disease process.

If preliminary tests of toxicity and efficacy indicate that the compound is worth advancing further, full-scale acute and chronic toxicity tests are carried out in animals. These include long-term tests of mutagenic or carcinogenic potential, effects on fertility, and teratogenicity. Mutagenicity tests may also be performed in microbial systems (Ames test).

Provided the animal toxicity studies reveal no serious toxicity problems, the first tentative trials are undertaken in healthy human volunteers to investigate the pharmacokinetic properties and safety of the new drug in man. Although animal data provide only a crude estimate of how the drug may be handled in human beings, if properly interpreted they allow an estimate to be made for the first human dose-ranging studies. Once these tests have been successfully completed, application may be made to the drug-licensing authority for permission to undertake clinical trials.

Clinical trials

The proof of the pudding is in the eating, and no amount of in-vitro or animal testing can replace the ultimate test of safety and efficacy: therapeutic use in human infection. Nevertheless, the clinical trial stage remains, in many ways, the least satisfactory aspect of the testing of any new antimicrobial drug. The reasons for this are not difficult to find: 'infection' is not a static condition in which therapeutic intervention produces an all-or-none effect. Many factors, such as mobilization of the patient's own immune response, drainage of pus, or treatment of an underlying surgical or medical condition, may crucially affect the response to therapy. The patient may improve subjectively, even though the antimicrobial therapy has demonstrably failed to eradicate the supposed pathogen; conversely, the patient's condition may deteriorate despite bacteriological 'success'.

Design of trials

Clinical trials should not be undertaken lightly. They are difficult to design, tedious to perform, and are fraught with ethical pitfalls. The conduct of the trial requires close supervision by a medical practitioner dedicated to the task, who needs to have the full support of reliable and motivated nursing and laboratory staff, together with well-informed and compliant patients. Before undertaking a trial, a detailed protocol should be drawn up, defining the conditions for which the new treatment is intended, the dosage regimens to be used, and the treatment with which it is to be compared. Participating laboratories should be consulted to ensure that full facilities are available for the monitoring of microbiological progress and the detection of adverse reactions. Licensing authorities require studies to conform to strict standards of good clinical practice and good laboratory practice.

Careful consideration should be given as to whether the trial should be open, single-blind (treatment known to the prescriber only), or double-blind (treatment randomly allocated in a fashion unknown to prescriber or recipient). In general, uncontrolled, open trials are unsatisfactory, except as preliminary indicators of safety and efficacy. They may also be used to gain information on the most appropriate dose of an agent. Controlled, double-blind trials are the most desirable scientifically, but are subject to ethical difficulties in that the prescribing doctor does not have full control over the patient's treatment. Whatever format is agreed, it is important that the new agent should be compared with current 'best practice' to avoid spurious claims of superiority. Placebo-controlled studies are normally acceptable only if adequate treatment is unavailable or controversial.

Ethical requirements

Ethical considerations need to be taken fully into account. The basic principles that should govern all research involving human subjects are embodied in the Declaration of Helsinki, which was adopted by the 18th World Medical Assembly in 1964, with subsequent revisions. In many countries, health authorities have ethical committees that monitor clinical trial protocols. The committee will need assurance that the safety of the new compound has been satisfactorily established and will wish to ensure that written informed patient consent is obtained from trial participants. It will also require adequate safeguards for the detection of unexpected adverse reactions and may have views as to whether a double-blind format, or a placebo control, is acceptable.

Statistical considerations

Many ambitious trials fail because insufficient numbers of patients are found to fulfil the criteria required for the study. Alternatively, the condition may be one (acute cystitis is a good example) in which the natural cure rate is so high, and the efficacy of standard treatment so good, that huge numbers would have to be examined to establish the superiority of a new agent, although it may be possible to determine efficacy. It is essential to be reasonably sure, before the trial starts, that sufficient patients can be recruited to satisfy statistical requirements. During the conduct of the trial, regular checks of relevant microbiological, haematological, chemical, and radiological parameters should be made. All findings should be fully documented as soon as the information is available, rather than attempting to glean information from the patients' notes retrospectively, after the trial is completed.

Drug licensing

Most countries have enacted some sort of legislation aimed at controlling the marketing of pharmaceutical products. In the US, federal regulations are administered by the Food and Drug Administration (FDA). Within the

European Union, a Committee on Proprietary Medicinal Products issues guidelines for harmonizing regulatory requirements among member nations. The European Medicines Evaluation Agency, based in London, co-ordinates drug licensing and safety throughout the European Union, although companies can still seek registration of their products by national regulatory authorities.

In the UK, executive powers are invested in government health and agriculture ministers, who constitute the Licensing Authority. Ministers are advised directly through the Medicines and Healthcare Products Regulatory Agency of the Department of Health. The Agency, through its specialist advisory committees, reviews all pharmaceutical products intended for medical or veterinary use. The licensing, manufacture, promotion, and distribution of all medicines intended for human use are supervised by the Commission on Human Medicines, which combines the functions of the Committee on Safety of Medicines and the Medicines Commission. The Commission acts as an independent agency in relation to particular issues and concerns, including any challenge to the decisions of the Licensing Authority.

Before clinical trials can be performed on a new drug in the UK, full toxicological data must be submitted to the Medicines and Healthcare Products Regulatory Agency together with a full trial protocol and the names of the proposed investigators. Such applications are scrutinized by the Committee on Safety of Medicines, who must satisfy themselves that all reasonable criteria are met before recommending that a clinical trial authorization should be issued. If the authorization is approved, investigators must undertake to notify any adverse reaction arising during the trial, or any other matter that might reasonably cause the Licensing Authority to doubt the safety or quality of the product.

When clinical trial data have been accumulated, an application for a marketing authorization (formerly called a product licence) may be made. All valid applications are again passed to the Committee on Safety of Medicines for scrutiny. In the UK new applications are judged solely on the grounds of safety, efficacy, and quality. If marketing authorization is refused, the application may be withdrawn or the applicant may elect to answer the objections raised, either in writing or in person before the committee. Should the application still be refused, the applicant has the right of appeal to the Medicines Commission. Marketing authorizations, once issued, are valid for 5 years in the first instance.

Over the years, the requirements of licensing authorities worldwide (particularly for toxicological testing) have become progressively more stringent.

Table 32.2 Antimicrobial agents (excluding topical agents) on the WHO model list of essential medicines (2005). Drugs shown in brackets, are on the complementary list

Antibacterial agents[a]	Antimycobacterial agents[a]	Antifungal agents	Antiviral agents — Antiherpes	Antiviral agents — Antiretroviral[a]	Antiprotozoal agents — Amoebiasis and giardiasis	Anthelminthic agents — Intestinal worms
Amoxicillin	Clofazimine	Clotrimazole	Aciclovir			
Ampicillin	Dapsone	Fluconazole[d]			Diloxanide[d]	Albendazole
Azithromycin[b]	Ethambutol	Griseofulvin			Metronidazole[d]	Levamisole
Benzathine penicillin	Isoniazid	Nystatin		Abacavir	**Leishmaniasis**	Mebendazole[d]
Benzylpenicillin	Pyrazinamide	(Amphotericin B)		Didanosine	Meglumine antimonate[d]	Niclosamide
Cefixime[c]	Rifampicin	(Flucytosine)		Efavirenz	(Amphotericin B)	Praziquantel
Chloramphenicol	Streptomycin	(Potassium iodide)		Indinavir	(Pentamidine)	Pyrantel
Ciprofloxacin[d]	(Amikacin)			Lamivudine	**Malaria[a]**	**Filariasis**
Cloxacillin[d]	(p-Aminosalicylic acid)			Lopinavir + ritonavir	Amodiaquine	Ivermectin
Co-amoxiclav	(Capreomycin)			Nelfinavir	Artemether + lumefantrine	(Diethylcarbamazine)
Co-trimoxazole	Cycloserine			Nevirapine	Chloroquine	(Suramin)
Doxycycline	(Ethionamide)			Saquinavir	Doxycycline	**Trematodes**
Erythromycin[d]	(Kanamycin)			Zidovudine	Mefloquine	Praziquantel
Gentamicin[d]	(Levofloxacin)				Primaquine	Triclabendazole

Table 32.2 (continued) Antimicrobial agents (excluding topical agents) on the WHO model list of essential medicines (2005). Drugs shown in brackets, are on the complementary list

Antibacterial agents	Antimycobacterial agents[a]	Antifungal agents	Antiviral agents	Antiprotozoal agents	Anthelminthic agents
Metronidazole[d]	(Ofloxacin)			Proguanil	(Oxamniquine)
Nitrofurantoin				Quinine	
Phenoxymethylpenicillin				(Artemether)	
Procaine penicillin				(Artesunate)	
Spectinomycin				(Sulfadoxine + pyrimethamine)	
Trimethoprim				**Trypanosomiasis**	
(Ceftazidime)				Benznidazole	
(Clindamycin)				Melarsoprol	
(Ceftriaxone[c])				Nifurtimox	
(Imipenem + cilastatin)				Suramin	
(Sulfadiazine)				(Eflornithine)	
(Vancomycin)				(Pentamidine)	

Data from the World Health Organization website: http://whqlibdoc.who.int/hq/2005/a87017_eng.pdf

[a]Most of the antimycobacterial, antiretroviral and antimalarial drugs are used in combination and many are available in fixed-dose combination preparations.

[b]For genital and ocular chlamydial infections only.

[c]For single-dose treatment of uncomplicated ano-genital gonorrhoea only.

[d]Examples of a therapeutic group for which acceptable alternatives exist.

mechanisms in some common pathogens. But the harsh truth is that the declining financial rewards available in this area have led pharmaceutical companies to divert many of their resources to the more lucrative field of antiviral and, to a lesser extent, antifungal compounds. Antiparasitic drugs remain grossly neglected, except for veterinary use.

Chemotherapeutic options for the treatment of non-bacterial infection remain very unsatisfactory. Although great strides have been made in the prevention of viral infection by immunization, and there have been important developments in antiviral agents, notably for the treatment of HIV infection, chemotherapy for viral disease is still extremely constrained (see Chapters 6, 7, and 27). Some sort of effective chemotherapy is available for most fungal, protozoal, and helminth infections, but the choice is very limited and, in many ways, unsatisfactory (see Chapters 4, 5, and 31). On a global scale these conditions are responsible for much of the morbidity and mortality from infectious disease that afflicts mankind. The greatest challenge for the future is to provide for these diseases the same sort of safe, effective chemotherapy that is now available for most bacterial infections, and to make effective therapy for all infections readily available for those who need it most.

Internet sites

Association of the British Pharmaceutical Industry. http://www.abpi.org.uk
British National Formulary. http://bnf.org/bnf
Electronic Medicines Compendium. http://www.medicines.org.uk
European Medicines Evaluation Agency http://www.emea.eu.int
National Institute for Health and Clinical Excellence. http://www.nice.org.uk
Scottish Medicines Consortium http://www.scottishmedicines.org
United Kingdom Medicines and Healthcare Products Regulatory Agency. http://www.mhra.gov.uk
United States Food and Drug Administration. http://www.fda.gov

Recommendations for further reading

General texts

Since the availability and use of antimicrobial agents vary widely in different countries, no one book has universal applicability. Among the most authoritative general texts in the English language are:

Bryskier A. *Antimicrobial agents—antibacterial and antifungals*. ASM Press, Washington, 2005.

Finch RG, Greenwood D, Norrby SR, Whitley RJ. *Antibiotic and chemotherapy: anti-infective agents and their use in therapy*, 8th edn. Churchill Livingstone, Edinburgh, 2003.

Kucers A, Crowe SM, Grayson ML, Hoy JF. *The use of antibiotics: a clinical review of antibacterial, antifungal and antiviral drugs*, 5th edn. Butterworth-Heinemann, Oxford, 1997.

An indispensable guide to the use of all therapeutic drugs for practitioners in the UK is provided by:

British National Formulary. British Medical Association and the Royal Pharmaceutical Society of Great Britain (revised twice yearly). Also available as an electronic version at http://bnf.org/bnf

Comprehensive monographs on antimicrobial agents are to be found in large reference texts on drugs including:

Dollery C (ed.). *Therapeutic drugs* (2nd edn). Churchill Livingstone, Edinburgh, 1999.

Sweetman SC (ed.). *Martindale: the complete drug reference* (34th edn). Pharmaceutical Press, London, 2004. (Also available online.)

Other useful texts on specific topics

Antiviral agents and the chemotherapy of viral infections

Butera ST (ed.). *HIV Chemotherapy: a critical review*. Horizon Bioscience, Norwich, 2005.

Challand R, Young RJ. *Antiviral Chemotherapy*. Oxford University Press, Oxford, 1997.

Driscoll JS. *Antiviral Drugs*. John Wiley & Sons, Chichester, 2005.

Galasso GJ, Whitley RJ, Merigan TC (eds.). *Antiviral Agents and Human Viral Diseases*, (4th edn). Lippincott, Williams and Wilkins, Baltimore, MD, 1997.

Diseases caused by protozoa and helminths (see also WHO publications below)

Aden Abdi Y, Gustafsson LL, Ericsson O, Hellgren U (eds.). *Handbook of Drugs for Tropical Parasitic Infection*, (2nd edn). Taylor and Francis, London, 1996.

Campbell WC, Rew RS (eds.). *Chemotherapy of Parasitic Diseases.* Plenum Press, New York, 1986.

James DM, Gilles HM. *Human Antiparasitic Drugs: pharmacology and usage.* Wiley, Chichester, 1985.

Rosenthal PJ. *Antimalarial Chemotherapy: mechanisms of action, resistance, and new directions in drug discovery.* Humana Press, Totowa, NJ, 2001.

Mode of action of antimicrobial agents and mechanisms of resistance

Franklin TJ, Snow GA. *Biochemistry and Molecular Biology of Antimicrobial Drug Action,* (6th edn). Springer-Verlag, New York, 2005.

Harrison J, Lederberg J (eds.). *Antimicrobial Resistance: issues and options.* National Academy Press, Washington, 1998.

Richman DD (ed.). *Antiviral Drug Resistance.* Wiley, Chichester, 1996.

Salyers AA, Whitt DD. *Revenge of the Microbes: how bacterial resistance is undermining the antibiotic miracle.* ASM Press, 2005.

Scholar EM, Pratt WB. *The Antimicrobial Drugs,* (2nd edn). Oxford University Press, New York, 2000.

Standing Medical Advisory Committee Report. *The Path of Least Resistance.* Department of Health/Public Health Laboratory Service, London, 1998.

Walsh C. *Antibiotics: Actions, origins, resistance.* ASM Press, Washington, 2003.

White DG, Alekshun MN, McDermott PF. *Frontiers in Antimicrobial Resistance. A tribute to Stuart B Levy.* ASM Press, 2005.

Laboratory methods

Lorian V (ed.). *Antibiotics in Laboratory Medicine,* (5th edn). Lippincott Williams & Wilkins, Baltimore, MD, 2005.

Reeves DS, Wise R, Andrews JM, White LO (eds.). *Clinical Antimicrobial Assays.* British Society for Antimicrobial Chemotherapy and Oxford University Press, Oxford, 1999.

Antibiotic resistance monitoring

Centers for Disease Control and Prevention, Atlanta, Georgia. Antibiotic/antimicrobial resistance. http://www.cdc.gov/drugresistance/index.htm

European Union: *European Antimicrobial Resistance Surveillance System.* http://www.earss.rivm.nl. The website has links to various national and international networks.

UK and Ireland: British Society for Antimicrobial Chemotherapy resistance surveillance. http://www.bsacsurv.org

Surveillance of antibiotic prescribing

European surveillance of antimicrobial consumption. http://www.esac.ua.ac.be/main.aspx?c=*ESAC2&n=21600. The website has publications from the project, which has collected and published data about community and hospital use of antibiotics across Europe from 1997. There are links to various national and international networks.

Learning resources about antimicrobial chemotherapy

The APT Project: appropriate prescribing for tomorrows' doctors. http://www.dundee.ac.uk/facmedden/APT/. The website has learning resources (clinical problems and prescribing exercises) created by medical schools in the UK with the aim of teaching prudent use of antibiotics in all clinical contexts.

WHO publications

The World Health Organization issues a wide variety of publications many of which are available on-line through the website http://www.who.int/. Of particular relevance to antimicrobial chemotherapy are:

Crompton DWT, Montresor A, Nesheim MC, Savioli L. *Controlling Disease due to Helminth Infections.* 2004.

Frieden T. *Toman's Tuberculosis. Case Detection, Treatment and Monitoring*, (2nd edn), 2004.
http://whqlibdoc.who.int/publications/2004/9241546034.pdf

Mehta DK, Ryan RSM, Hogerzeil H. *WHO Model formulary.* 2004.
http://mednet3.who.int/EMLib/wmf.aspx

WHO Essential Drug Monitor. http://www.who.int/medicines/publications/monitor/en

WHO Global malaria programme. http://malaria.who.int

WHO Global strategy for containment of antimicrobial resistance.
http://www.who.int/drugresistance/en/

WHO Guidelines for the treatment of malaria. http://www.who.int/malaria/docs/TreatmentGuidelines2006.pdf

WHO Model Prescribing Information: *Drugs used in parasitic diseases*, (2nd edn). 1995.

WHO. *TB/HIV: a clinical manual*, (2nd edn). 2004. http://www.who.int/tb/publications/who_htm_tb_2004_329/en/index.html

Journals

Papers dealing with aspects of the use of antimicrobial drugs appear in numerous journals. English language journals specifically devoted to antibiotics and antimicrobial therapy include:

Antibiotics and Chemotherapy
Antimicrobial Agents and Chemotherapy
Antiviral Chemistry and Chemotherapy
Antiviral Research
Chemotherapy
International Journal of Antimicrobial Agents
Journal of Antibiotics
Journal of Antimicrobial Chemotherapy
Journal of Chemotherapy.

Index